THE 5ᵀᴴ ARTICLE OF THE ORDINANCE OF CONGRESS OF 1787

WISCONSIN MEDICINE
Historical Perspectives

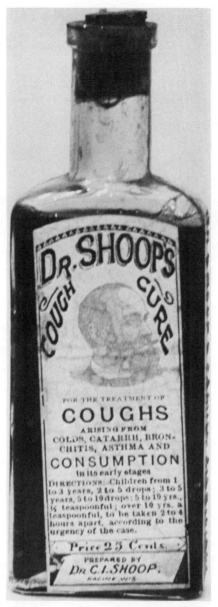

Patent medicines, like Dr. Shoop's Cough Cure, bottled in Racine, offered Wisconsin residents a popular alternative or supplement to professional medical care.

Wisconsin
Medicine
Historical
Perspectives

Edited by
Ronald L. Numbers
and
Judith Walzer Leavitt

THE UNIVERSITY OF WISCONSIN PRESS

Published 1981

The University of Wisconsin Press
114 North Murray Street
Madison, Wisconsin 53715

The University of Wisconsin Press, Ltd.
1 Gower Street
London WC1E 6HA, England

First printing

Printed in the United States of America

For LC CIP information see the colophon

ISBN 0-299-08430-2

endpaper map: 1839 map of "Wiskonsin" territory, compiled from the public surveys, courtesy of the State Historical Society of Wisconsin, WHi (X31)17448

To the memory of
William Snow Miller (1858–1939)
and
William Shainline Middleton (1890–1975)
Pioneers of the History of Medicine in Wisconsin

Contents

Acknowledgments ix

Introduction 3

1. Frontier Medicine in the Territory of Wisconsin
Peter T. Harstad 13

2. From Horse and Buggy to Automobile and Telephone:
Medical Practice in Wisconsin, 1848–1930 Guenter B. Risse 25

3. Sectarians and Scientists: Alternatives to Orthodox
Medicine Elizabeth Barnaby Keeney,
Susan Eyrich Lederer, and Edmond P. Minihan 47

4. Public Protection and Self-Interest: Medical Societies in
Wisconsin Ronald L. Numbers 75

5. From Infirmaries to Intensive Care: Hospitals in
Wisconsin Philip Shoemaker and Mary Van Hulle Jones 105

6. One Hundred Years of Health and Healing in Rural
Wisconsin Dale E. Treleven 133

7. Health in Urban Wisconsin: From Bad to Bet
Judith Walzer Leavitt 155

8. A Note on Medical Education in Wisconsin
Ronald L. Numbers 177

Selected Sources on the History of Medicine in
Wisconsin Deanna Reed Springall 185

Contributors 201

Index 203

Acknowledgments

This volume originated with a Bicentennial symposium, "Wisconsin Medicine, 1776–1976," sponsored by the Department of the History of Medicine, University of Wisconsin–Madison, in cooperation with the Charitable, Educational and Scientific Foundation of the State Medical Society of Wisconsin. For financial assistance with publishing costs, we wish to thank the following: the University of Wisconsin Medical School and Associate Dean Ralph A. Hawley, a longtime friend of the history of medicine; the Charitable, Educational and Scientific Foundation of the State Medical Society and its president, Robert T. Cooney, M.D.; the William Dorrence Memorial Fund; and the Department of the History of Medicine, University of Wisconsin–Madison.

WISCONSIN MEDICINE
Historical Perspectives

Introduction

Most people, if they think about the subject at all, associate Wisconsin's medical history with the digestive experiments William Beaumont performed on a man with a hole in his stomach. They know nothing about the less dramatic, but even more consequential, developments in the state's medical annals. Thanks to advances in medicine, public health, nutrition, and hygiene, life expectancy at birth has nearly doubled since territorial days.[1] During the same period the physician has risen from a position of marginal respectability to one of unparalleled admiration and trust. The hospital, unknown to residents 150 years ago, has become a symbol of modern science and a source of civic pride. Knowledge of disease has revolutionized health practices.

The purpose of this volume is not to celebrate the achievements of Wisconsin's physicians, notable as they have been, but to look critically and sympathetically at the state's medical record. The contributors make no exaggerated claims for Wisconsin. Occasionally it led the nation in matters of health, but more often it followed the example of others. Our goal is to understand how and why Wisconsin's medical practice evolved and to illuminate the processes by which change occurred.

On epidemiological and cultural grounds, a regional or local approach might be more logical than a state history. In their fascinating

study of *The Midwest Pioneer: His Ills, Cures & Doctors*, Madge E.
Pickard and R. Carlyle Buley discovered not only a common medical
history in the Midwest, but also "a distinct spirit of regional self-
consciousness."[2] Other historians have preferred to restrict their attention to individual cities, whose populations, though neither ethnically
nor economically uniform, shared numerous local experiences.[3] Despite
the methodological appeal of regional and urban studies, we have decided to focus our attention on the state, the traditional unit of study for
historians of American medicine. This tradition dates back to the nineteenth and early twentieth centuries, when a number of historically
minded physicians sought to immortalize their predecessors.[4] The first
generation of professionally trained medical historians continued the
tradition, beginning with John Duffy's *History of Medicine in Louisiana* in 1958 and Thomas N. Bonner's *Kansas Doctor* the following year.[5]

Although diseases knew no state lines and cultural attitudes toward
sickness transcended political boundaries, state activities markedly
influenced medical history. State licensing laws determined the qualifications of health-care professionals, state charters and universities controlled medical training, state boards of health promoted hygienic standards and combated disease, state institutions housed the mentally and
physically ill, and other state agencies regulated such activities as medical insurance, nursing homes, and the sale of drugs. Thus state histories
of medicine, despite their obvious limitations, can reveal developments
that regional and local histories tend to overlook.

This brief history of health care in Wisconsin, admittedly traditional
in scope, is unique in one respect. For the first time, to our knowledge, a
group of professional historians representing several specialties has collaborated on writing the medical history of a state. This arrangement
meant giving up the unity and comprehensiveness of single-authored
volumes, but we believe the gains in diversity and depth have been
worth the sacrifice.

Medical history in Wisconsin began thousands of years ago with the
arrival of the first American Indians from Asia. Little is known about
pre-Columbian medical practices, although archeologists working in
the Great Lakes area have discovered suggestions of medico-religious
rituals and traces of medicine bundles.[6] When the first white men visited present-day Wisconsin in the seventeenth century, they found an
estimated 20,000 Indian people, mostly Fox, Sauk, Kickapoo, Mascouten, Miami, Winnebago, Menominee, Potawatomi, Chippewa, and
Ottawa. Although some, like the Winnebago, had long resided in the
area, many others had only recently come to the western side of Lake
Michigan.[7]

Both archeological and historical testimony suggests that Wisconsin's indigenous inhabitants suffered few of the contagious diseases that had long plagued Europeans and to which the latter had built up a degree of immunity. Jonathan Carver, who explored the upper Mississippi Valley in the 1760s, reported that "The Indians in general are healthy, and subject but to few diseases . . . that afflict civilized nations." The Indian population did, however, suffer greatly from war, exposure, and hunger; and Carver found cases of pleurisy ("the disorder to which they are most subject"), dropsy, and paralysis.[8]

The arrival of Europeans and their diseases brought disaster to the American Indians. Infection spread rapidly from tribe to tribe, sometimes striking even before the first contact with Europeans. Measles, influenza, and venereal diseases felled countless victims, but smallpox proved to be the deadliest of all. Dr. Douglass Houghton, who vaccinated hundreds of Chippewa in 1832, found them to "have a wonderful dread of the Small Pox." He estimated that this disease had struck at least five times since the 1760s. During the 1832 smallpox epidemic the Potawatomi reportedly "died off like sheep," and a subsequent outbreak two years later killed approximately one quarter of the Winnebago, who "fled before it like a stricken deer, leaving their dead and dying behind them."[9]

Healing practices varied markedly from tribe to tribe and changed with the passage of time, but certain similarities existed. Central to an understanding of American Indian medicine is a recognition of the intimate relationship between religion and medicine. Although the Indian people attributed minor cuts and bruises to natural causes, they typically viewed serious illness as resulting from an offense to one of the many spirits who inhabited the world around them or from the malevolent actions of another human. Thus, as the anthropologist Richard I. Ford has stressed, discovering *who* caused the illness became the first and most important task of the Indian healer.

The Indian doctors, who diagnosed and treated the sick, combined the roles of doctor, priest, and magician. These healers, who enjoyed high social status, often specialized in particular forms of therapy. Conjurers, for example, used their clairvoyant powers to discover the cause of sickness and to effect magic cures, while sucking doctors magically removed disease-causing foreign objects. Women often served as midwives, herbalists, and bone-setters; after menopause they were eligible to practice medicine like men.

Therapy depended on the nature and cause of the particular illness. To treat common complaints, the people of the upper Mississippi Valley employed a great variety of practical herbal remedies, including emetics, laxatives, febrifuges, and coagulants, which they administered in the form of poultices, teas, and enemas (using a deer bladder connected to a bird bone or hollow reed). To relieve various aches and pains, they bled, tattooed, and scarified with sharp pieces of flint. But "their grand remedy," according to Carver, was the sweat bath — followed by a plunge into the nearest stream. Medicine men prescribed this form of hydrotherapy for persons suffering from colds, fevers, and rheumatism, frequently combining it with healing ceremonies.

Such ceremonies, which appealed to the spirits for relief or assistance, typically involved special dances, incantations, prayers, rattles, or drums, all orchestrated by a medicine man. One Winnebago prayer went as follows:

To you, grandmother, the Earth, I too offer tobacco. You blessed me and promised to help me whenever I needed you. You said that I could use all the best herbs that grow upon you, and that I would always be able to effect cures with them. Those herbs I ask of you now, and I ask you to help me cure this sick person. Make my medicine powerful, grandmother.[10]

Many Indian doctors reportedly enjoyed great success.

Until the late seventeenth century, when French voyageurs began invading the land between the upper Mississippi and Lake Michigan in search of furs, the American Indians had Wisconsin virtually to themselves. The arrival of European fur traders — first French, then British — severely disrupted the region's economy and ecology, but scarcely increased its population. When the United States government assumed control of Wisconsin at the conclusion of the War of 1812, it inherited, besides thousands of hostile Indians, only two villages, Green Bay and Prairie du Chien, with a combined population of a few hundred whites. To protect its interests, the United States quickly set up forts at these two locations and later added a third at Portage. The fort hospitals and their staffs brought Wisconsin its first European-style health care.

Close on the heels of the United States Army came thousands of miners, eager to exploit the lead deposits that lay along the western portion of the present Illinois-Wisconsin border. By 1836, when Wisconsin achieved territorial status, 11,683 whites were living in the territory east of the Mississippi. Nearly half of these people resided in the southwestern mining communities, the largest of which was Mineral Point. Milwaukee was a two-year-old hamlet, and Madison existed only on paper. Within a few years farmers and speculators were pouring into the territory, often entering through the port of Milwaukee after traveling along the Erie Canal and crossing the Great Lakes. Between 1836 and 1840 the territory's population grew by 164 percent; the following decade it increased nearly tenfold.

According to local boosters, no place offered better prospects for health. Wisconsin, declared one propaganda pamphlet, "is remarkably free from those causes of endemic diseases . . . which have been the misfortune of large portions of Michigan, and the scourge of Indiana, Illinois, Missouri, and part of Iowa. Wisconsin is conceded to be the healthiest of western States."[11] Unrestrained by such modesty, Milwaukee's Increase Lapham wrote in 1844 that "our most intelligent physicians" believe "that Wisconsin is, and will continue to be, one of the most healthy places in the world."[12] Such words gave comfort to prospective settlers, who feared the prospect of sickness and premature death more than anything else.

The very year Lapham penned his praise, however, a recent Norwegian immigrant told a different story of life in the Territory of Wisconsin.

The first thing we encountered on our arrival in Milwaukee was two of our countrymen down at the wharf. Not until then did we see the good things one acquires in this country — an emaciated body and a sallow face! This is how almost all our immigrants look. The ague and other pestilential fevers were widespread so that one victim could not help the other. All who have this illness become weak, are never safe from it, and daily suffer from poor health. . . . Except for a few men, all are in misery from illness, starvation, and cold.[13]

Unfortunately for those who settled in Wisconsin, the Norwegian's experience proved all too typical.

Throughout the early decades of settlement no disease took a greater toll than malaria, commonly called ague. Along the mosquito-infested waterways favored by early residents, there was virtually no escape. During the summer of 1830 over three-fourths of the men stationed at low-lying Fort Crawford in Prairie du Chien came down with malaria.[14] Although most victims survived, death was not uncommon. In 1841 malaria killed 80 of the 600 residents of Lake Muskego; and before the disease declined in the last third of the century, annual death rates from malaria ran as high as 5.7 per 10,000.[15]

Pioneers who survived malaria faced a host of other health hazards. In addition to occasional outbreaks of deadly cholera and smallpox, they contended with widespread typhoid fever, dysentery, and erysipelas — to say nothing of childhood diseases like scarlet fever, measles, and diphtheria.[16] To compound their troubles, they received little help from the medical profession, which knew almost nothing about the cause of disease and even less about its cure. Any man brazen enough to call himself "doctor" could practice with impunity, and many did. Under such circumstances it is not surprising that early residents often chose to treat themselves or suffer in silence.

The second half of the nineteenth century brought rapid change to Wisconsin. Between 1850 and 1900 its population swelled from about 300,000 to over 2,000,000, while the percentage of city dwellers increased from 9.4 to 38.2. By the end of the century Milwaukee alone, now a major commercial and industrial center, claimed 285,315 inhabitants, many of them European immigrants.[17]

With the increase in population came corresponding changes in health conditions and medical care. The incidence of malaria decreased markedly as the railroads, which arrived in the 1850s, carried settlers away from the mosquito-infested river valleys and as farmers drained their lands, turned to dairying, and built better houses. Illness, however, continued to plague Wisconsin residents, who increasingly fell victim to tuberculosis, dysentery, and typhoid fever.[18] Milwaukee — filthy, smelly, and congested — suffered the most. But in 1867, inspired by the recent success of New York City's Metropolitan Board of Health, the city created a board of health to fight disease by cleaning the streets, providing pure water, and disposing of waste. By 1910 Milwaukee ranked among the seven American cities with the lowest death rates, and two decades later the American Public Health Association designated it the healthiest large city in the United States. For the first time in Wisconsin history, the city was as safe as the farm.

The influx of immigrants into Milwaukee led to the creation in 1848 of Wisconsin's first nonmilitary hospital, St. John's Infirmary. Such institutions, however, did not become widespread until the last decades of the century, when anesthesia and antisepsis (later asepsis) popularized hospital surgery. By 1900 over 50 general hospitals and 25 mental hospitals were serving Wisconsin residents.

The rise of the hospital, together with the advent of the telephone and the automobile, revolutionized the practice of medicine. Unlike pioneer physicians, who had generally practiced in the homes of their patients, early twentieth-century doctors worked largely in hospitals or in their own offices, where patients came to them. These changes benefited patients as well as doctors: they facilitated access to professional medical care by allowing physicians to treat more patients per day and reduced costs by eliminating charges for time on the road.[19]

The second half of the nineteenth century also witnessed a therapeutic revolution, as the excessive bleedings and purgings of territorial days gave way to specific medications and vaccines. An array of new medical instruments and laboratory techniques permitted unprecedented diagnostic precision and brought scientific respectability to the profession. Nevertheless, it was long after neighboring states had established medical examining boards and four-year medical schools that Wisconsin belatedly rewarded its physicians with a medical licensing law and a two-year medical college.

The concentration of both population and medical care in centers around the state has characterized the period since the First World War. In the 1920s, for the first time in the history of Wisconsin more residents lived in cities than in the country, and a disproportionate number (roughly one in four) crowded into the highly industrialized southeastern corner of the state. At the same time medical technology and patient needs accelerated the fragmentation of the medical profession into a multitude of specialities, and the popularity of group practices eroded the position of the solo practitioner. To deal with the complexities of modern medicine, doctors in such places as Marshfield, La Crosse, and Madison began collecting into clinic-based groups; by the 1920s Wisconsin led the nation in such organizations. These multi-specialty clinics and the growing number of sophisticated hospitals brought first-class medical care to virtually every region of the state and no doubt assisted in reducing mortality, especially among newborn infants. But they also contributed to the overriding concern of health planners during the late twentieth century: the increasingly high cost of medical care.

Although the essays in this volume add significantly to our knowledge of medicine in Wisconsin, large gaps remain. Physicians, for example, dominate the pages of this book; yet they never monopolized medical care in the state. In addition to many allied health professionals such as dentists, optometrists, podiatrists, psychologists, pharmacists, nurses, and midwives, there have been countless quacks and folk healers and millions of individuals who treated themselves. These healers are mentioned only in passing, if at all. Their stories — and many more — deserve to be told, and it is our hope that this collection will serve as a foundation for further research, not as a capstone to the efforts of the past.

Notes

1 Judith Walzer Leavitt and Ronald L. Numbers, eds., *Sickness and Health in America: Readings in the History of Medicine and Public Health* (Madison: University of Wisconsin Press, 1978), p. 4.
2 Madge E. Pickard and R. Carlyle Buley, *The Midwest Pioneer: His Ills, Cures, & Doctors* (New York: Henry Schuman, 1946), p. 199. Peter T. Harstad reached a similar conclusion in "Health in the Upper Mississippi River Valley, 1820 to 1861" (Ph.D. diss., University of Wisconsin, 1963), p. v.
3 Midwestern examples include Thomas N. Bonner, *Medicine in Chicago, 1850–1950: A Chapter in the Social and Scientific Development of a City*

(Madison: American History Research Center, 1957), and Judith Walzer Leavitt, *The Healthiest City: Milwaukee and the Politics of Health Reform* (Princeton: Princeton University Press, forthcoming).

4 Among the Midwestern contributions to this genre are G. W. H. Kemper, *A Medical History of the State of Indiana* (Chicago: American Medical Association Press, 1911); C. B. Burr, ed., *Medical History of Michigan*, 2 vols. (Minneapolis: Bruce Publishing Co., 1930); Lucius H. Zeuch, ed., *History of Medical Practice in Illinois: Preceding 1850* (Chicago: Book Press, 1927); and David J. Davis, ed., *History of Medical Practice in Illinois: 1850–1900* (Chicago: Illinois State Medical Society, 1955).

5 John Duffy, ed., *The Rudolph Matas History of Medicine in Louisiana*, 2 vols. (Baton Rouge: Louisiana State University Press, 1958, 1962); Thomas Neville Bonner, *The Kansas Doctor: A Century of Pioneering* (Lawrence: University of Kansas Press, 1959). Philip D. Jordan's earlier volume, *The People's Health: A History of Public Health in Minnesota to 1848* (St. Paul: Minnesota Historical Society, 1953), focused on preventive rather than curative medicine.

6 Richard I. Ford, "Health Views and Practices among Early Wisconsin Indians," unpublished paper presented in March 1976 at a Bicentennial symposium, "Wisconsin Medicine: 1776–1976," sponsored by the Department of the History of Medicine, University of Wisconsin–Madison. The following description of healing practices among the Wisconsin Indians is based on Ford; Virgil J. Vogel, *American Indian Medicine* (Norman: University of Oklahoma Press, 1970); Robert E. Ritzenthaler, "Chippewa Preoccupation with Health: Change in a Traditional Attitude Resulting from Modern Health Problems," *Bulletin of the Public Museum of the City of Milwaukee* 19 (1953): 175–258; Harold Hickerson, *The Chippewa and Their Neighbors: A Study in Ethnohistory* (New York: Holt, Rinehart and Winston, 1970), Chapter 4; and J[onathan] Carver, *Travels through the Interior Parts of North America, in the Years 1766, 1767, and 1768* (facsimile ed.; Minneapolis: Ross & Haines, 1956), pp. 384–95. We would like to thank Nancy Oestreich Lurie, of the Milwaukee Public Museum, for her helpful suggestions.

7 Robert C. Nesbit, *Wisconsin: A History* (Madison: University of Wisconsin Press, 1973), p. 12; William C. Sturtevant, ed., *Handbook of North American Indians*, Vol. 15: *Northeast*, ed. Bruce G. Trigger (Washington: Smithsonian Institution, 1978), pp. 594–601, 636–786.

8 Carver, *Travels*, pp. 389–91.

9 Quotations from Alice E. Smith, *The History of Wisconsin*, Vol. 1: *From Exploration to Statehood* (Madison: State Historical Society of Wisconsin, 1973), p. 100.

10 Paul Radin, *The Winnebago Tribe* (Lincoln: University of Nebraska Press, 1970), p. 227, quoted in Ford, "Health Views and Practices."

11 Quoted in Harstad, "Health in the Upper Mississippi River Valley," p. 42.

12 Increase A. Lapham, *A Geographical and Topographical Description of Wisconsin* (Milwaukee, 1844), p. 91, quoted in Harstad, "Health in the Up-

per Mississippi River Valley," pp. 39–40. See also Pickard and Buley, *Midwest Pioneer*, p. 15.

13 Quoted in Harstad, "Health in the Upper Mississippi River Valley," p. 321.

14 Smith, *History of Wisconsin*, p. 99.

15 Erwin H. Ackerknecht, *Malaria in the Upper Mississippi Valley, 1760–1900* (Baltimore: Johns Hopkins Press, 1945), pp. 44–48.

16 Erwin H. Ackerknecht, "Diseases in the Middle West," in *Essays in the History of Medicine* (Chicago: for the Davis Lecture Committee, by the University of Illinois Press, 1965), pp. 168–81.

17 Nesbit, *Wisconsin*, pp. 342, 548.

18 Ackerknecht, "Diseases in the Middle West."

19 Paul Starr, "Medicine, Economy and Society in Nineteenth-Century America," in *The Medicine Show*, ed. Patricia Branca (New York: Science History Publications, 1977), pp. 47–66.

1 *Peter T. Harstad*

Frontier Medicine
in the Territory of Wisconsin

Frontier medicine evokes an image of a doctor mounting his steed and galloping off into the night on an errand of mercy. Anxious friends beckon him into a dimly lit log cabin to escort a new citizen through "the triumphal arch of civilization," to set a broken bone, or to assert in hushed tones that death is near and mortals can do nothing to forestall it. Such scenes reveal only one side of frontier medicine, but they took place frequently enough to help establish a model of the doctor-patient relationship that has outlived the frontier physician, his mode of transportation, and the usefulness of nearly all the medicines he carried in his saddlebags. Although frontier medicine persisted in some parts well into the twentieth century, nearly all the material in this chapter pertains to the Territory of Wisconsin, which existed, chronologically, from 1836 to 1848.

During an Independence Day celebration at Mineral Point in 1836, Henry Dodge took the oath of office to become the first governor of the Territory of Wisconsin, a vast expanse including all of the present states of Wisconsin and Iowa and portions of Minnesota and the two Dakotas. As head of the newest political subdivision of the United States, Dodge ordered a census, which enumerated 11,683 white people living in four counties east of the Mississippi River and 10,531 whites residing in Dubuque and Desmoine counties west of the great river. Disease and death

13

were not strangers to these early settlers. As Governor Dodge observed in one of his addresses to the Legislative Assembly of the Territory of Wisconsin: "The lot of the settlers on the public lands has been one of hardship, privation and toil, exposed alike to the dangers of savage warfare, and diseases incident to the settlement of a new country."[1]

Among the many threats to life and health in the territory none was more serious than malaria (also called ague), a fact that often surprised visitors from the East. When approaching Burlington in 1837, the year the territorial assembly met in that Mississippi River town, a concerned Yankee mother spotted two children on the bank who had crawled out from a hut "into the warm sun with chattering teeth to see the boat pass." They were the "most pitiable looking objects, uncared for, hollow eyed, sallow-faced." With an eye to her own offspring the mother raised a series of questions to which the captain replied:

If you've never seen that kind of sickness I reckon you must be a Yankee; that's the ague. I'm feared you'll see plenty of it if you stay long in these parts. They call it here the swamp devil, and it will take the roses out of the cheeks of those plump little ones of yours mighty quick. Cure it? No madam. No cure for it; have to wear it out. I had it a year when I first went on the river.[2]

The symptoms were unmistakable: periodic chills, fever, sallow cheeks, sunken eyes, enlarged spleen, and general lack of energy. Nevertheless, many settlers along the water courses in southern Wisconsin came to regard malaria, not as an illness, but as an inevitable part of the "acclimatization" process for newcomers. As one pioneer said of another, "He ain't sick, he's only got the ager."[3]

During the early years of Fort Crawford (at Prairie du Chien), Fort Winnebago (at Portage), and Fort Howard (at Green Bay), malaria constantly plagued the United States Army. According to the *Statistical Report on the Sickness and Mortality in the Army of the United States* (1840), a compilation of thousands of quarterly reports, 72 percent of the men stationed at Fort Crawford during the third quarter of 1830 suffered from malaria. Like most of his contemporaries, the fort surgeon, William Beaumont, better known for his experiments on digestion, attributed the cause to "marsh miasmata."[4]

At least twice during the 1840s the famous Ohio Valley physician Daniel Drake visited the Territory of Wisconsin to study the etiology of malaria. During one of his trips, probably in 1842, he learned from a "respected Indian trader" living near Fort Howard that malaria was unknown in Green Bay before 1828. From his own data and from military reports Drake concluded that, despite a few cases of malaria, the environment around Fort Howard was generally salubrious.[5]

On another occasion, possibly a year or two later, Drake traversed the southern part of the territory, from Milwaukee to Galena, again recording the factors that might be contributing to malaria. In the vicinity of the Four Lakes (Madison) he thought that he might have reached a latitude at which climate may be supposed "in some degree, to overrule topographical conditions, in the production of autumnal fever." As was his habit, Drake quizzed local medical practitioners and learned from a Dr. Weston of Madison that malaria had appeared in the town and that there had been one sickly season.[6]

In his massive *Treatise . . . on the Principal Diseases of the Interior Valley of North America* (1850) Drake explored the relationship between malaria and the environment around Fort Winnebago. Despite being located near the "shaking" marshes common to the region between the headwaters of the Fox and Wisconsin rivers, a topography "eminently" favorable to malaria, Fort Winnebago experienced a lower incidence of the disease than Fort Howard. Noting that the former occupied land a degree farther south but 225 feet higher in altitude than the latter, Drake hypothesized that the difference in altitude more than compensated for the difference in latitude. He thus concluded that "a latitude of forty-three degrees and a half, and an elevation eight hundred feet, greatly control the noxious autumnal influence of extensive bogs and marshes, abounding in organic matter."[7]

Drake went on in this book to speculate that malaria was caused by "living organic forms, too small to be seen with the naked eye, and which may belong to either the vegetable or animal kingdom, or partake of the characters of both." He termed this speculation his "vegeto-animalcular hypothesis."[8] How close to the mark he was and yet how far from identifying the malaria parasite and its carrier, the Anopheles mosquito.

If the residents of the Territory of Wisconsin gradually lost their fear of endemic health hazards like malaria, they remained terrorized by the threat of imported infections. The very devil himself could hardly have designed a better carrier for harmful microorganisms than the fast steamboats that plied the Mississippi River, its major tributaries, and Lake Michigan. The heaviest traffic and most crowded conditions came during the warmest months, when conditions were most favorable to disease transmission. Deck passengers ate at the same mess, drank surface water from common dippers, and dried themselves on public towels. Wisconsin's major settlements were regular ports of call for steamboats and frequently points of dispersal for communicable diseases.

The Territory of Wisconsin escaped the most feared scourge of all, Asiatic cholera, only because this disease was not present in the United

States or the Western world during Wisconsin's twelve years as a territory. Just before and immediately after these years cholera raged unrestrained through the region. During the Black Hawk War of 1832,
when cholera posed a greater threat to life than the Indians, Henry
Dodge had ordered that "every soldier or Ranger who shall be found
drunk or sensibly intoxicated . . . (shall) be compelled, as soon as his
strength will permit, to dig a grave at a suitable burying place, large
enough for his own reception, as such grave cannot fail soon to be
wanted for the drunken man himself, or some drunken companion."[9]
Unfortunately, neither Dodge's order nor the advice of the best medical
men of the day proved valuable in controlling the lethal cholera bacillus.

When Wisconsin broke off from Michigan Territory in 1836 to become a separate territory, it inherited the laws that had governed the
old political unit. The most important statute pertaining to health, a
bill passed in response to the 1832 cholera epidemic, empowered officials to inspect vessels, to detain or isolate persons infected with "pestilential disease," and to require the cleansing of houses or outhouses
"likely to endanger the public health."[10] An 1833 Michigan act set rudimentary standards for the measuring and packing of foodstuffs, requiring, for example, that some grades of salt pork not contain legs, ears,
snouts, or "faces."[11] Also applicable to the Territory of Wisconsin was a
law preventing anyone from practicing physic or surgery "until he shall
have passed examination" from a medical society incorporated under
terms detailed elsewhere in the act. This smacked of monopoly, a concept contrary to the prevailing winds of Jacksonian Democracy. The
act clinched the suspicion of special privilege by stipulating that doctors
who would not submit to the above process were "forever . . . disquali-
fied from collecting any debt or debts, incurred by such practice, in any
court in this territory."[12] It appears that Henry Dodge, true to the
philosophy of Andrew Jackson, who appointed him governor, took no
part in the enforcement of this or any similar act. Along with most of his
fellow citizens, he believed that government had no rightful role in
matters of individual health — except when punishing criminals or wag-
ing war.

The first session of the Wisconsin territorial assembly did, however,
pass one piece of legislation relating to health. A section of a bill on the
incorporation of towns empowered local officials "to present and remove nuisances, . . . to regulate and establish markets, to open ditches,
and to provide for drawing off water, to sink and keep in repair public
wells." Governor Dodge apparently refused to sign the bill.[13]

In 1847, the year before statehood, a legislative committee noted that
the regular practice of medicine, "consisting of the general features of

bleeding, purging, vomiting, and injections, cataplasms, blisters, poultices and leeching," had lately been "invaded by a tribe of interlopers, who, without license and without lancets, under the various names of homoeopathists, hydropathists, animal magnetizers, phreno-magnetizers, urine doctors, and poudrette doctors, undertake to cure our diseases without any regular system, purging us chiefly of our substance, and bleeding our pockets more than our veins." According to one politician, the committee contemplated a law "subjecting such offenders to be operated on by their own systems, and to swallow their own medicines." Legislation seemed unwise, however, after one faction began advocating the suppression of all species of quackery — including quack lawyers and quack politicians.[14]

One of the best-trained regular physicians in the territory was Dr. Thomas Steel, whose career reveals much about the practice of frontier medicine at mid-century. Born into a middle-class Scottish family in 1809, he began his college education at the University of London and received his M.D. from the University of Glasgow in 1833. After wide travels in North America and the Orient, the young doctor continued his studies at Paris, the leading medical center of the Western world. For a half-dozen years he tried with meager economic success to practice medicine, dentistry, or a combination of the two in London. But the late 1830s and early 1840s were depressed and troubled years. It bothered Dr. Steel that even as a bachelor he could not support himself without assistance from his father.[15]

In 1843 Dr. Steel fell in with some disciples of Robert Owen in a London coffeehouse. A score of these Londoners soon set their hearts on communal living on a farm in the Territory of Wisconsin. They needed a physician and convinced Steel, healthy, adventuresome, and always a bit of a radical, to sign up as physician to the Society of Equality. Before the year was out the Equalitarians resided on their own lands on the borders of Spring Lake, not far from Mukwonago. "This part of the country is rapidly settling," Steel wrote to his father in London on September 9, 1843. "There is no doctor within a large extent of country and our neighbors all express themselves delighted that a doctor has come amongst them — and my friends have taken every opportunity of blazing my fame to the skies, so that I have no doubt I will have a good deal to do by and bye."

In a matter of weeks Steel came to feel that his affiliation with the Society was detrimental to his interests: the Society agreed to purchase a horse to enable him to make professional calls in the surrounding community; in return, Steel was to deposit all of his earnings in the Society's general fund. Steel's statement that not one of the Equalitarians was

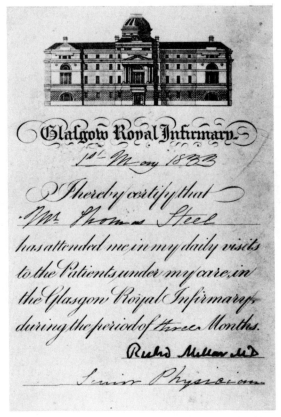

Before immigrating to Wisconsin, Thomas Steel spent three months on the wards of the Glasgow Royal Infirmary in Scotland.

"prepared for any other state of society than the one they have left" applied to himself. He left the Society, bought some land, and went into private practice. In exchange for a supply of medicines, Steel agreed to administer to the health needs of the Equalitarians for a period of six months. Upon the expiration of this contract, a rare and early arrangement for dealing with matters of health in a collective way came to an end in youthful Wisconsin.

Since his patients were scattered and he could not buy a horse immediately, Steel traveled great distances on foot. "I wish you could see me setting out on my professional visits," he wrote on December 13, 1843, "with my big boots made of cow hide coming up to the knee over my trousers. You would admit that I am becoming Yankyfied fast." With

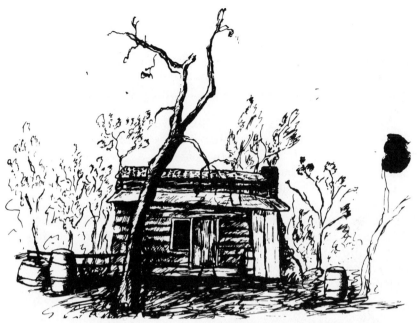

State Historical Society of Wisconsin, WHi(X3)36712

In a letter to his father, Dr. Thomas Steel sketched the cabin in which he first stayed after settling in present-day Waukesha County.

no professional rivals in the immediate area, prospects looked good for the young doctor.

The disease Steel treated most frequently was malaria. Steel was so fortunate in his treatments that he "got the name of the doctor who cures the disease slick off," he wrote home proudly on November 13, 1843. "This character I mainly deserve from the circumstance of my having brought with me from London some good *Sulphate of Quinine*, a medicine not to be procured genuine in this part of the country." During his early years in Wisconsin, Steel begged his father to send such articles as quinine, morphine, smallpox vaccine, as well as medical books, lancets and other instruments.

In lieu of cash for his services and medicines, Steel frequently accepted produce, animals, or farm labor from the families of his patients. To take advantage of such assets, Steel felt compelled to go into farming. He built a farmstead about a mile north of Spring Lake and for the first time in his adult life put down some roots. He married an Equalitarian woman and together they began raising a family not far from the village of Genesee. Had it not been for the labor of his wife's

family and the periodic Bank of England notes from his father, the
Steels could not have enjoyed any of the niceties of life during the territorial period, and at times they would have been short of necessities.
From August 1846 through July 1847, Steel earned an average of $20.85
a month including the value of goods and services received. From this
must be deducted the cost of his quinine and other drugs and also the
cost of keeping his horse.[16]

Practicing medicine on the agricultural frontier was sporadic and exhausting work. It was not an unusual day when Steel traveled thirty
miles on horseback to visit only two patients. As roads became better,
he used a small carriage and, in the winter, a light sleigh.

Generally, Steel visited the sick in their homes. When a situation became critical he spent hours and even days at a patient's bedside. Ordi-
narily, he was not called into maternity cases unless complications
developed. On one occasion in 1844 Steel used his "every exertion" to
save the life of a woman in childbirth "during eight days, in which time
I never had my clothes of[f]." After consulting with a Prairieville (Waukesha) physician, Dr. Gilbert Wright, Steel removed a fetus piece by
piece, in the presence of all the old women of the neighborhood.[17] In
this instance the patient died. It was Steel's custom to attend the funer-
als of his patients.

Like many doctors of the period, Steel frequently functioned as a
dentist. In one of his early letters from Wisconsin, he wrote that he expected to "get a job now and then in the teeth way." News of his skill at
pulling teeth quickly spread. When people came to him for an extrac-
tion, the charge was fifty cents; "when sent for one dollar." Steel soon
noticed that several farmers' wives and daughters had artificial teeth. "I
was asked today by a lady as to how much I would charge for supplying
her with three fronts," he wrote on December 2, 1843. The settlers also
requested filling and scaling. By the end of the territorial period a few
practitioners in the larger towns devoted full time to dentistry, an early
specialization in medical practice.

Although Dr. Steel was for the most part isolated from men of his
education and experience, he read medical journals and books and on
occasion attended meetings of medical societies. For example, on May
5, 1846, he attended the organizational meeting of the Milwaukee
County Medical Society, "where I met with about fifteen Physicians."
He explained to his father in London in a letter of May 15:

The law authorizes the Medical men in each county to form a society, for their
mutual protection, also for the purpose of examining the qualifications of candidates for the Medical profession. For the present there is to be an annual sub-
scription of one dollar, two meetings yearly for non-attendance upon which a

fine of one dollar is to be exacted. After settling the business, i.e. adopting the laws, electing the president and vice president &c. the Town Physicians invited those from the country to dinner at the City Hotel. We had a pretty good dinner, two glasses of beer each & coffee, but no wine spirits or toast drinking. I left the same evening, slept on the road and next morning reached home where I found all well.

Steel attended the 1847 annual meeting of the organization, but the only other references to Steel in the Society's Minute Book concern delinquency of assessed fees and fines for nonattendance of meetings. In 1848, when a number of Wisconsin doctors pushed for special privileges in the law for collection of their debts, Steel criticized them in the public press.

At the end of the territorial period, with five years of medical practice in Wisconsin behind him, Steel perceived "a great want of principle amongst the men practicing medicine here, generally running each other down in the most unprincipled manner." The English and Scotch continued to be his steady friends, "but the Yankies are fond of change, and have not quite so high a standard of morals as the others, so are apt to judge others by themselves." Steel claimed to be more successful among the English and Scotch because they confided in him and heeded his advice. "Amongst the Yankies," he noted, "you are watched suspiciously, your mode of treatment criticized, and your advice probably altogether neglected in conformity with their ideas of independence." Steel asserted: "I have more than once taken my hat and walked of [f], advising them to get some other assistance."[18] He might have added that those suspicious Yankee eyes sometimes fell on the well-used bloodletting instruments in his bag.

At times, being a frontier doctor was "a harassing occupation to mind and body."[19] With the benefit of hindsight we can see that the limits of medical knowledge, the expectations of neighbors and loved ones, and the rigors of working conditions combined to place heavy burdens on the early medical practitioners of Wisconsin — burdens men like Steel did not share with hospitals, clinics, or other medical institutions. The only exception to this would be an occasional consultation with a neighboring physician. Perhaps to escape his burden, in 1881 Steel left the community where he was known so well and moved to Milwaukee.

How did Steel bear up in comparison with those who qualify as his peers? Quite well, it seems. Prior to Steel's arrival in Wisconsin in 1843, only one "regular" physician, Gilbert Wright, resided in what became Waukesha County. Wright "sustained domestic trouble," took to alcohol and drugs, became demented, and died in the public poorhouse in 1891. Dr. Henry A. Youmans settled in the county the same year Steel

came and died there fifty years later after an active career in medicine
and public life. Dr. Jeremiah Youmans practiced with his brother,
Henry, at Mukwonago, but died of "general paralysis" at the State Hospital for the Insane in 1873. Dr. William Griffith, a young British physician who seems to have stepped into Steel's practice in the late 1870s,
became addicted to alcohol and morphine, and was institutionalized
for insanity for a time before his death in 1903. Thus, out of this group
of five practitioners, only Steel and Henry Youmans escaped serious
mental derangement. Steel, who died in 1896, outlived all his professional peers except Griffith, a much younger man.[20]

Notes

1 John Porter Bloom, ed., *The Territorial Papers of the United States*, Vol. 27
(Washington: Government Printing Office, 1969), p. 132. For population
figures, see ibid., p. 84.

2 Quoted in Truman O. Douglass, *The Pilgrims of Iowa* (Boston: Pilgrim
Press, 1911), p. 25.

3 Quoted in Erwin H. Ackerknecht, *Malaria in the Upper Mississippi Valley,
1760–1900* (Baltimore: Johns Hopkins Press, 1945), p. 5.

4 Bruce E. Mahan, *Old Fort Crawford and the Frontier* (Iowa City: State Historical Society of Iowa, 1926), Ch. 9.

5 Daniel Drake, *A Systematic Treatise, Historical, Etiological and Practical,
on the Principal Diseases of the Interior Valley of North America, as They
Appear in the Caucasian, African, Indian, and Esquimaux Varieties of Its
Population* (Cincinnati: W. B. Smith & Co., 1850), pp. 337–39.

6 Ibid., pp. 328–29.

7 Ibid., pp. 339–40.

8 Ibid., p. 723.

9 Quoted in Louis Pelzer, *Henry Dodge* (Iowa City: State Historical Society of
Iowa, 1911), pp. 69–70.

10 *Acts Passed at the First and Second Sessions of the Legislative Assembly of
the Territory of Wisconsin* (Burlington: W. T. James Clarke, 1838), "Appendix, Containing a Number of the Most Important Laws of Michigan, Extended over the Territory of Wisconsin by the Act of Congress Organizing
Said Territory," pp. 268–69.

11 Ibid., pp. 231–37.

12 Ibid., pp. 261–66.

13 Ibid., pp. 51–55.

14 Moses M. Strong, *History of the Territory of Wisconsin, from 1836 to 1848*
(Madison: Democrat Printing Co., 1885), pp. 547–48.

15 The entire section on Dr. Thomas Steel is based upon items in the Steel Collection at the State Historical Society of Wisconsin, Madison, Wis.

16 Thomas Steel to James Steel (his father), August 1, 1847.

17 Thomas Steel to James Steel, December 12, 1844.
18 Thomas Steel to James Steel, February 9, 1848.
19 Thomas Steel to James Steel, September 10, 1852.
20 Material on Steel's peers is drawn from county histories; *Waukesha Free-man*, February 19, 1891, and January 15, 1903; census data; and miscellane-ous sources at the Waukesha County Historical Society.

2 *Guenter B. Risse*

From Horse and Buggy to Automobile and Telephone: Medical Practice in Wisconsin, 1848–1930

Dr. William H. Washburn accurately assessed Wisconsin's place in national medicine when he commemorated the state medical society's seventy-fifth anniversary in 1921:

Medical practice in Wisconsin during the past 75 years has undoubtedly been typical of medical practice everywhere during that period. We have had our leaders and followers, our self-assertives and our modest, retiring and devoted physicians. . . . In times of stress and crises we have rendered our service both to mankind and to the state, and to the Nation, as have our confreres in sister states.[1]

Although typical of medical activities elsewhere in the Midwest, the story of Wisconsin physicians deserves to be told. It constitutes a vital chapter in the gradual evolution of American medicine from frontier heroics to applied science.

This chapter focuses on the curative activities of "regular" or "orthodox" physicians in the period between statehood and the Great Depression. In medicine these eighty-odd years witnessed the most radical transformation in theory and practice since the days of Hippocrates in ancient Greece. Three overlapping generations of Wisconsin physicians practiced during this period, each confronting different patterns of diseases whose changing incidence, puzzling transmission, and often confusing clinical features were closely related to the land, climate, human organization, and influx of new microorganisms. Poorly drained land favored malaria, better farm technology multiplied accidents, and urban crowding spawned smallpox, diphtheria, typhoid fever, and tuberculosis.[2]

Physicians applied theoretical knowledge learned from textbooks or assimilated through apprenticeships. Depending on whether they adhered to an antiphlogistic or stimulating system of medicine, they believed fevers could be starved or fed. Socioeconomic forces and technological advances also shaped medical practice, shifting its locus from home to office, dispensary, or hospital. During the early twentieth century the use of the telephone and automobile revolutionized medical practice by greatly expanding its scope and setting.

The Horse-and-Buggy Doctor: 1850–1890

When John Mitchell gave his presidential address at the state medical society's meeting in Madison on January 31, 1856, he purposely touched on one of the most crucial issues confronting contemporary medicine: lack of trust. "Perhaps no profession, art or even trade are looked upon with as much distrust as that of medicine," he declared. "Even prevailing schemes of quackery [i.e., the medical sects] are more highly esteemed by a majority of the people of many districts."[3]

Lack of public confidence and the absence of state licensing laws produced an uncertain status for physicians. The regular physicians who settled Wisconsin's frontier competed — often unsuccessfully — with botanical or steam doctors, homeopaths and hydropaths, as well as a variety of self-appointed quacks and drug peddlers who sold their wares through colorful advertisements. "There is nothing in which our newspapers are so well united as the puffing of quackery," concluded Mitchell indignantly.[4]

There was enough disease in Wisconsin to keep every healer busy, whether regular or sectarian. Malaria remained endemic in the Mississippi valley until the 1870s. Cholera epidemics swept through the state in 1849, 1866, and again in 1873. The lack of sanitary facilities greatly aided the spread of typhoid fever in villages and cities, while smallpox constantly menaced urban areas and lumber camps. The greatest and most constant toll of human lives, however, came from a variety of intestinal and respiratory ailments, labeled dysentery and pneumonia, which were especially fatal to infants.[5]

The horse-and-buggy doctor based his practice on knowledge essentially unchanged since the early 1800s. Outmoded views of vitality and disease stubbornly persisted, and reformers sporadically spoke out against "raw" empiricism. For many practitioners medical education still consisted of a few years of apprenticeship with an already established practitioner. Apprentices received room and board while learning medicine. In return, they often hitched up the team, drove the physician around to house calls, and took care of the horses. They also worked around the house, helping with repairs and filling patients' prescriptions. A few fortunate students supplemented such training with lectures in anatomy, pathology, and materia medica at one of the numerous medical schools outside Wisconsin.[6]

The pioneer physician depended on his senses for making a diagnosis. Percussion and auscultation with the aid of a stethoscope did not become widespread until late in the century.[7] Pulse and the characteristics of the tongue remained the mainstays of diagnosis as well as prognosis. The clinical thermometer was still a stranger to the black bag.

Wisconsin physicians treated most fevers with an array of drugs designed to assist nature in the removal of some bodily excesses or corruptions. Bleeding, vomiting, and purging the patient were standard therapeutic techniques. When vigorously applied in the presence of severe illness, they constituted the so-called "heroic" treatments largely responsible for patient distrust and apprehension.

Physicians bled most patients either by cutting a vein with a lancet or by extracting smaller amounts with the aid of scarificators and cups. They drugged patients with an assembly of unstandardized and evil-tasting powders, extracts, and tinctures: epsom salts, calomel, and jalap to purge the bowels; opium or its tincture, laudanum, to relieve pain; quinine to reduce fever; ipecac and tartar emetic to induce vomiting; and a combination of opium, ipecac, and antimony known as Dover powder to generate sweat.[8]

An example of this "heroic" practice is furnished by the 1856–58 diary of a Jefferson County practitioner, Dr. Horace B. Willard. During this time he treated a three-year-old boy for an intestinal ailment, using the purgative calomel, a potentially toxic mercurial preparation, together with rhubarb extract every three hours for the first days. Then he administered ipecac, a powerful emetic, and blistered the child to divert bodily corruptions from the innards to the skin. Fortunately, the patient recovered two weeks later in spite of ailment and treatment.[9]

Surgery was similarly rudimentary. In the absence of antiseptic methods, most rural and urban accidents involving fractures meant amputation — and a fee of $25 to $100.[10] The alternative was sepsis and gangrene. Chloroform sometimes alleviated surgical pain. As early as 1856 the state medical society at its annual meeting organized a presentation on the subject of anesthetic agents.[11]

The contemporary limitations of surgery were reflected in Horace O.

Crane's statistics from 1863–1865. A Green Bay practitioner and one of Wisconsin's nine medical examiners of recruits for the Civil War, Crane rejected 48.5 men per thousand for hernias and 12.5 for fractures and dislocations.[12] In spite of the circumscribed capacity of surgery to solve problems, the public expected competence. In one account from the 1850s a physician attending a wealthy patient with a leg fracture feared the possibility of a malpractice suit if his treatment did not accomplish the desired results.[13]

Early physicians also extracted teeth for 25 cents, using the dreaded "turnkeys." For $10 they attended deliveries shunned by midwives, employing forceps in difficult cases. They reduced hernias and anal prolapses, treated dislocations and fractures, dressed wounds, and opened abscesses.

A pioneer Wisconsin physician was on call twenty-four hours a day, seven days a week, throughout the entire year. Commonly, he would get up between 4 and 6 o'clock in the morning, feed his team of horses, and clean the mud-spattered buggy. After a hearty breakfast, he was off to make house calls. He traveled either on horseback, in a horse-drawn buggy, or, occasionally, on foot. He carried saddlebags containing the necessary surgical instruments, bandages, and drugs, plus an obstetrical case.[14]

Depending on weather and road conditions, he rode at a speed of two to five miles per hour to patients generally scattered within a twenty to twenty-five mile radius. During the winter physicians rode sleighs or cutters, prone to overturn in high snow drifts. Dr. J. V. Stevens of Sauk City carried a scoop shovel, axe, and wire cutter at all times. He often shoveled through drifts to fences along the road, cut them down, and proceeded to drive his sleigh through the fields.[15]

The rides required special precautions during Wisconsin's winters: fur coats and caps with earflaps, heavy mittens, felt boots, and the famous buffalo robes. Cutters kept a semblance of warmth through the use of heated soapstones or small charcoal stoves.[16] Some physicians rode specifically marked circuits between adjacent towns, such as Newman C. Rowley's daily trip from Middleton Depot to Mazomanie, Mt. Horeb, and Paoli,[17] or William H. Fox's route between Fitchburg, Oregon, and Stoughton.[18]

For all their exhausting travels, most pioneer physicians working in the rural areas earned a meager income. John C. Reeve, settling during the 1850s in a small Dodge County town, took in a mere $68 during his first year in practice.[19] A sample fee bill, issued in 1849 by the Western Medical Society of Wisconsin, charged $1 for visits in town, $2 for country visits under two miles, and an additional charge of 50 cents per mile

---

A. T. BLACKBURN, M. D.

—DEALER IN—

DRUGS *AND* MEDICINES

wall Paper and Jewelry, Toilet Articles and Stationery.

PRESCRIPTIONS CAREFULLY COMPOUNDED.

WALDO, - - WISCONSIN.

Wright's Directory of Sheboygan County for 1889–90, p. 308
(State Historical Society of Wisconsin)

Because of a surplus of physicians in the late nineteenth century, many practitioners, like Waldo's Dr. A. T. Blackburn, combined medicine with some other business.

beyond that. Bleeding was done for 50 cents, cupping for $1.[20] An 1844 Milwaukee fee bill quotes similar figures.[21]

Most patients did not pay their medical bills in cash. For example, in Spring Green during the 1880s they paid a quarter of beef for a pneumonia case, a $5 pig for a normal birth, and several hams for minor surgery.[22] A 50-cent office visit brought three haircuts, half a duck, eight dozen eggs, a bushel of potatoes, or seven pounds of cheese.

An important part of Wisconsin medical practice was the care of lumberjacks and sawmill workers in the northern "piney" counties. The lumber business topped the list of Wisconsin manufacturers until 1910 and provided one fourth of all state wages. From the early period of settlement to the late 1880s, the lumbering industry attracted large numbers of young and adventurous people, who were exposed to hazardous, unhygienic living and working conditions. A transient and rowdy labor force, the self-reliant lumberjacks treated some of their chilblains, knifing wounds, and upper respiratory infections themselves. Smallpox, typhoid fever, and severe work accidents often required the services of "Quinine Jimmy" or "Epsom salts," as the visiting physician was known in lumberjack lingo.[23]

Because of the remote location of most camps, physicians' visits were expensive. For example, Marinette physicians charged $5 for a call to the Peshtigo Harbor Camp, and most workers, making $26 to $30 a month, could not afford the fee. In 1885 three Marinette physicians entered into an agreement with the Peshtigo Company, agreeing to furnish medical care to all employees at a rate of $1.25 per month for married men and their families and 75 cents per month for single men. The company deducted these fees from the men's pay.[24] This prepaid medical care was supplemented by a hospital insurance program designed by the Marinette and Menominee Hospital Company to provide care for the very ill at the hospitals in both cities. Loggers could buy hospital tickets for $5, entitling them to hospitalization for one year, including medical and surgical services.[25]

After the Civil War, returning military physicians improved surgery in Wisconsin. As early as 1870 the committee on surgery of the state medical society reported the use of carbolic acid in four cases.[26] The subsequent popularity of antiseptic methods prompted Dr. John Favill of Madison to declare enthusiastically in 1872 that "surgery in some departments is rapidly approaching perfection."[27]

Wisconsin's leading surgeon, Nicholas Senn, presented an important paper on bone necrosis the same year.[28] This condition, which had hitherto prompted immediate and generous amputations, was now preventable through the application of antisepsis. Improved plaster-of-Paris bandages became available during 1874, making prolonged bed confinement for fracture cases no longer necessary. The use of air pumps to aspirate infectable body fluids accumulating at the site of incisions and wounds greatly decreased the morbidity associated with surgical interventions.[29]

Senn, who practiced in Milwaukee for twenty years before moving to Chicago, was an acknowledged world leader in gastric and intestinal surgery.[30] He helped bring new European advances and discoveries to the attention of Wisconsin physicians. In 1881, while serving as chairman of the state medical society's committee on surgery, he spoke optimistically of a "complete revolution in surgery."[31] Antiseptic surgery was not, however, customary in country practice. Many rural surgical procedures omitted proper antiseptic techniques. Family wash boilers helped to clean towels and instruments. Dr. S. S. Riddell of Chippewa Falls insisted that it was "almost impossible to carry the antiseptic machinery along" when making house calls. And Dr. E. F. Dodge of Fond du Lac wondered why "should one incumber oneself with all the paraphernalia used by Lister if proper cleanliness could guarantee similar results."[32] Potentially acute abdominal afflictions continued to suffer from lack of careful and frequent follow-up, especially when the calls involved ten to fifteen mile trips under adverse weather conditions.[33]

Changes in diagnosis and therapy occurred rapidly after 1870. Wisconsin physicians employed stethoscopes and thermometers, ophthalmoscopes and laryngoscopes.[34] The impact of early bacteriology was not far behind. "The relation of microorganisms to disease is the most important question before the medical profession today," noted Dr. J. S. Walbridge of Berlin, Wisconsin, when chairman in 1883 of the committee on practice.[35] The germ theory of disease gradually gained new adherents, and its implications for diagnosis and pathology became more visible. "The pathology of the future will reap in this field its most fertile and profitable harvest," prophesied Senn.[36] With the help of microscopes, some practitioners began to examine blood smears and urine sediments, thus achieving greater diagnostic as well as prognostic precision.

A perusal of the state medical society's *Transactions* reveals a quiet revolution in therapeutics. Physicians ceased to treat infectious diseases with depleting measures. They restricted bloodletting to convulsions in puerperal eclampsia and to strokes.[37] Patients suffering from typhoid fever received salicylic acid or antipyrine, a German product discovered in 1884.[38] Nitroglycerine was introduced in 1876 for the treatment of angina pectoris, and chloral hydrate became recognized as an effective sedative.[39]

Physicians frequently denounced the bulky and nauseous drugs of yesteryear; instead, single and active agents were recommended. In 1881 James G. Meachem, Jr., chairing the state medical society's committee on new remedies, declared that 50 percent of the contemporary remedies had been introduced in the preceding three decades. Improved chemical and pharmacological knowledge led to specific drug action, smaller doses, and palatable compounds. "Emulsions, elixirs, tasteless pills, capsules, wafers and compress tablets — all nice to take — now cover the nauseous taste and vile odors that helped to 'kill or cure' thirty years ago," reported Meachem. "Now it is sugar and spice, and all things nice, under the cover of the aromatics."[40]

These changes in medical practice were significant enough to brand most mid-century practitioners "old fogies, who prefer to finish life's course by moving along in the same time-worn rut of thought and habit."[41] One doctor concluded: "There are but few practitioners except in sparsely settled districts, who have the hardihood to stride the leather pill bags, or drive the one-horse shay of a quarter of a century ago. Such a rig would now attract as much of a crowd as a traveling menagerie."[42] By 1890 in Wisconsin an era had ended.

Years of Transition: 1890–1910

Wisconsin physicians in the 1890s were optimistic about their future. Prevailing health conditions, however, did not yet reflect the benefits of the new medicine. Smallpox and tuberculosis were rampant. Mortality rates remained high. The fearful conditions led the governor of Wisconsin to make an unusual offer in 1891: "I am prepared tonight to offer a premium of one million dollars to the specialist or any other man

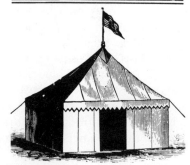
To help physicians combat tuberculosis, the leading cause of death in the early twentieth
century, Joys Brothers of Milwaukee sold tents for consumptive patients.

who will produce in the State of Wisconsin a cure for diphtheria."[43]

Although nobody ever collected the governor's bounty, Loran Beebe
of Superior treated his young patients with diphtheria antitoxin from
Germany shortly after it became available.[44] In 1895 the Milwaukee
Health Department distributed antitoxin to the various diphtheria stations around the city.[45] Two years later Dr. William Whyte of Watertown presented the first paper in Wisconsin on the successful treatment
of laryngeal diphtheria with the new antitoxin.[46] Gradually the hitherto life-saving intubation and tracheotomy procedures were abandoned
in favor of serotherapy. Within ten years the mortality rate from this
childhood scourge fell by half. Armed with diphtheria antitoxin, tetanus antitoxin (1894), and the antimeningococcic serum (1907), physicians began impressing the public with their therapeutic efficacy.[47]

Asked to recall the most salient diagnostic improvements of the period,
a Janesville physician named the sphygmomanometer for the measure-
ment of arterial blood pressure, an instrument invented by Riva Rocci
in 1896. Lumbar punctures were initiated in 1891 to carry out chemical
and bacteriological studies on the spinal fluid, especially in meningitis.

Beginning in 1896 the Widal agglutination reaction was used in the diagnosis of the still-dreaded typhoid fever.[48] Improvements in the lens and lighting of the cystoscope facilitated urological diagnostic and surgical procedures.

Very soon after Roentgen's discovery of the X rays in 1895, a Milwaukee pharmacist, Jacob S. Janssen, obtained the first radiographic exposure in Wisconsin and constructed a portable X-ray unit for use in Milwaukee hospitals.[49] As Janssen recalled later, he took radiographs requiring exposure times of more than forty-five minutes. Not understanding the dangers of radiation, he lost one hand and several fingers of the other.[50] As early as 1902 Milwaukee physicians were employing Roentgen rays therapeutically to treat breast cancer.[51]

The newer diagnostic techniques, the expansion of minor surgical procedures, and the increased mobility of patients in urban settings gradually shifted a fair portion of medical practice to the physician's office. Increased use of offices allowed physicians more time with patients. But many complained that office practice was convenient only to doctors. Governor Peck grumbled in 1891: "The old physician covered more territory than the whole medical society today if they stay in their offices."[52]

Offices had reception and consultation rooms, working quarters that doubled as laboratories, pharmacies, and emergency rooms. A Waukesha practitioner kept in his office his journals, a winter's supply of wood, and an iron hospital cot for convenient afternoon catnaps.[53] William Osler thought the most powerful professional tool of this period was "the little laboratory room attached to the office of the general practitioner."[54] With more complicated office practices, physicians began to keep records of clinical and financial information and some observers began advocating business training for medical students.[55] A few specialists employed business managers or bill collectors.

Aseptic surgery became popular in the 1890s. The techniques to exclude pathogenic germs from the operating field required fastidious preparations such as the sterilization of instruments, sutures, dressings and aprons, and the careful scrubbing of the patient's skin near the incision.[56] The new approach required extra cleanliness from the physician. "A surgeon who carries the odor of iodoform with him does not know how to wash his hands," declared one Wisconsin surgeon.[57] One well-known surgeon believed tobacco smoke was a sterilizing and disinfecting agent. He lit his cigar before going into the operating room and smoked it throughout the surgical procedure.[58] Most practitioners, while consenting to wear butchers' aprons, still did not wear caps, masks, or gloves. "The whiskers died hard," commented William C. Ground of Superior, "and as they were considered a sign of virility, the doctors like everyone else were reluctant to give them up. Surgically they were clearly a menace, and before mowing them down completely, they were placed in a bag which the nurse would more or less deftly tie around the surgeon's head."[59]

The newly gained confidence in surgery led to demands from people for knife-assisted solutions to their troubles. The patient's first question became "Doctor, can't you cut it out?" observed F. W. Epley in 1896.[60] Ovariotomies cured everything from backaches to insanity; hysterectomies and appendectomies were very frequent. One Milwaukee practitioner reflected that surgery was beginning to fall into discredit because of "much reckless and very unnecessary operating."[61]

The improvements in surgery created tension between general practitioners and specialists. Family physicians in the smallest towns felt obliged to adopt some specialty. "It takes no prophet to foresee that if present conditions increase, family physicians will become as extinct as the ichthyosaurus, and ere long suffering humanity will be treated by a syndicate of physicians," lamented one.[62] By the turn of the twentieth century Wisconsin physicians were genuinely worried about the effects of fragmented care of patients.[63]

Aided by the increased practice of surgery, medical practice increasingly shifted to hospitals. Home kitchen tables gave way to small operating rooms. As C. R. Bardeen pointed out, general hospitals were chiefly developed in response to the demands of surgeons for proper facilities.[64]

The telephone, in common use by the end of the century, changed medical practice almost as much as the hospital. It allowed patients to communicate rapidly with their physicians, and it permitted doctors to follow up their cases without time-consuming house calls and to summon consultants in difficult cases. But it also created problems. After installing a telephone in his office, Dr. Marcus Bossard of Spring Green found himself on the road more often than before, responding to patient calls.[65] Other physicians complained about the frequent interruptions when the phone rang.[66] According to an editorial in the *Wisconsin Medical Journal*, "Long distance holdups of this character are increasing in frequency as the popularity and number of telephones increase."[67] Because of the bother, many physicians charged ordinary office fees for giving telephone advice.

Malpractice litigation became a common concern in the 1890s. H. B. Favill singled out two factors to explain the increasing number of suits: the physician's failure to discharge his obligations to the public and the public's inability to appreciate the position of the physician. Clinical conditions were always approximate, variable, and inferred, and these characteristics had to be communicated to the patients.[68] "In no countries are malpractice suits as prevalent as in the United States and Britain," noted one Wisconsin physician, who criticized physicians for publicly speaking out against other physicians and patients for threatening malpractice suits to get a discount.[69]

Increased competition among practitioners with varying skills and widely diverging educational backgrounds lay at the root of the difficulties between doctors and their patients. "It cannot be denied that there is manifest within our profession an increasing tendency to purely commercial methods," said a Sheboygan physician in 1899; "its inevitable results must be misunderstanding, discord and ill-feeling."[70]

The state medical society in 1907 established a committee to study the question.[71] A Milwaukee practitioner, Armin Mueller, asserted that except for cases of obvious wanton carelessness, all malpractice suits were the result of insinuations or instigations of other physicians, whom he characterized as "shyster" doctors. Mueller urged the unceremonious expulsion of such doctors from the medical society, with the long-term objective of closing ranks within the profession.[72]

At its next meeting the council of the society approved a plan for "Medical Defense." It became the duty of the society's executive committee to investigate all claims of malpractice filed against its members. If a case could be properly defended, the society's attorney assisted the accused physician.[73] The adoption of the Medical Defense plan was hailed as a pivotal move toward increasing professional harmony and prosperity.[74]

Looking back on the transitional decades between 1890 and 1910, J. M. Dodd of Ashland provided a mixed review. On the positive side, Dodd acknowledged the impressive successes of public health and medical science. He stressed the elimination of overzealous, symptomatic therapeutics and nauseating, nonessential remedies. Yet, declared Dodd, "a commercial spirit is invading our profession to an alarming degree, leading to questionable methods to obtain practice, such as commissions, divisions of fees and lodge practice."[75] Thus, paradoxically, while the advances of scientific medicine allowed the elimination of previous scourges such as smallpox, cholera, and yellow fever, as well as the amelioration of diphtheria, typhoid fever, and tuberculosis, the general public continued its criticisms of the profession.[76]

The Gasoline Era: 1910–1930

New legal regulations affected Wisconsin practitioners in the second decade of the twentieth century. The 1911 Occupational Diseases Act required physicians to report cases of poisoning from lead, phosphorus, arsenic, mercury, or their compounds. The so-called Eugenics Law of

1913 obligated physicians to issue premarital certificates to all males, attesting to their freedom from venereal diseases. Another law the same year made fee-splitting a criminal offense. Finally, the national Harrison Narcotic Act of 1914 created control mechanisms for the prescription and dispensation of narcotic drugs.

Despite these new regulations, public distrust of the medical profession lingered.[77] The resultant frustrations of the medical profession largely evaporated, however, during the First World War. As in other parts of the country, repeated appeals were made to Wisconsin physicians for establishing a Medical Reserve Corps.[78] Although not all responded to the appeal, more than 30,000 physicians volunteered nationwide, accepting commissions. The medical profession believed that such an expression of patriotism was bound to find favor with the public. In 1918 the president of the state medical society seemed to recognize a new national mood when he declared: "Momentous changes have taken place within the past year and a half in the attitude of the public toward the medical profession. . . . [It] is one of the greatest, most valuable assets the country possesses in its great struggle for universal liberty."[79]

The health conditions uncovered in military recruits disturbed physicians. Forty percent of the volunteers between the ages of 21 and 30 were declared unfit to serve. Chronic otitis, pulmonary tuberculosis, spinal deformities, and valvular heart disease stemming from rheumatic fever were seen as conditions resulting from insufficient prophylactic measures.[80] Physicians also uncovered a high incidence of syphilis: 1.2 percent of all Wisconsin recruits suffered from the disease. In spite of the availability of the Wassermann test after 1906, uncertainties in diagnosis and expensive, protracted treatment stifled medical efforts to control the problem.[81]

Just as the Civil War had influenced Wisconsin medical practice, so too did the First World War. Because of the success of team work in the Army Medical Corps, group practice was brought home to civilian settings.[82] Wisconsin played a leading role in the development of this important innovation in medical practice.[83] One of the most successful group practices was started in 1916 by six physicians in Marshfield, a central Wisconsin community of 3,400 people. Marshfield provided an ideal setting for such a venture, with a well-equipped hospital and an able, congenial group of physicians. The clinic was staffed by two surgeons, a radiologist, an internist, an ophthalmologist, and a urologist. The growth of the Marshfield Clinic was impressive. In 1920 a total of 23,329 patients were seen in the clinic's offices.[84] In La Crosse, two Norwegian physicians, Adolf Gundersen and Christian Christensen, formed another flourishing group practice.[85] In Madison the pioneer surgeon James H. Jackson, Sr., joined with his four physician sons to establish the Jackson Clinic in 1917. By 1922 the medical staff had grown to ten practitioners, including Arnold S. Jackson, the well-known "goiter surgeon."[86]

In his 1920 presidential address to the state medical society, Charles R. Bardeen praised the advantages of organized medical clinics.[87] By 1922 Wisconsin led the nation in the number of group clinics, followed closely by Minnesota. That year the American Medical Association expressed support for group practice on the grounds that it afforded efficient specialized care and supported the general practitioner with consultations.[88]

The generation of physicians graduating after the implementation of the educational reforms stemming from the Flexner Report of 1910 dramatically increased the accuracy of diagnosis and scored the first triumphs of chemotherapy.[89] While the major focus of practice remained in the area of acute infectious diseases, a gradually aging population with their degenerative ailments posed further diagnostic and therapeutic challenges. Modern diagnosis relied heavily on X rays and the clinical laboratory. Comprehensive blood and urine examinations, analyses of other body fluids, and bacteriological methods were increasingly employed.[90] Serological tests such as the typing of pneumococci and meningococci, blood grouping and matching, and the new Kolmer quantitative complement fixation test for syphilis became available. Chemical analysis of the blood, especially the determination of urea, creatinine, uric acid, and sugar, helped to ascertain the presence of metabolic diseases.

On the therapeutic front, biological treatment and prophylaxis with antitoxins, serums, and vaccines remained prominent. Antistreptococcus and antipneumococus sera proved disappointingly ineffective, forcing physicians merely to continue their previous expectant attitude.[91] The advent of arsphenamine, discovered in Germany by Paul Ehrlich, signaled the beginnings of modern chemotherapy. Its widespread use after 1910, as a compound specifically toxic to spirochetes, enabled physicians to expect a cure in syphilis.[92]

Another major therapeutic breakthrough came with the discovery in 1921 of insulin for the treatment of diabetes. A year later some Wisconsin physicians were already employing this life-saving pancreatic extract.[93] A variety of other organ extracts — notably thyroid, ovarian, testicular, and adrenal — were used for endocrine disturbances.

The increased reliance on laboratory medicine coupled with the needs of aseptic surgery expanded the role of hospitals in medical practice. The decade after the war witnessed the most dramatic growth of hospitals in Wisconsin, with the addition of 65 new institutions, about 30 percent of the total. At the same time, many of the previously established hospitals expanded and modernized. By 1930 Wisconsin had 225 registered hospitals with a capacity of 24,393 beds, representing one bed for every 277 inhabitants, a figure close to the national average. Hospitals had truly become, in Charles R. Bardeen's view, indispensable instruments in the modern practice of medicine.[94]

The automobile further affected medical practice after the war. Beginning in the mid-1890s, physicians increasingly seized this mode of transportation to expand their practices. In some cases doctors virtually tripled their number of house calls.[95] There were other advantages. As one physician noted: "The automobile and the telephone have set people's minds at rest. They don't send for me in the middle of the night the way they used to . . . now they know I can get there in no time if needed, and they do not worry."[96]

The early automobiles were not easy to handle, especially in Wisconsin winters. Open touring cars without heaters or defrosters often tested the stamina and ingenuity of their owners. Physicians persisted despite the difficulties, and by the 1920s effects of the automobile were evident. The expansion and extension of medical services accentuated the com-

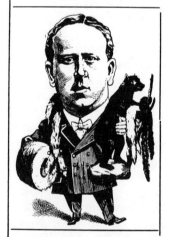
Wisconsin Medical Journal 6 (1907–8): xxxix

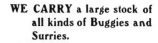
Wisconsin Medical Journal 5 (1906–7): xxxi

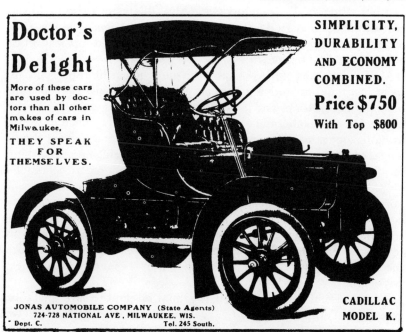

Wisconsin Medical Journal 5 (1906–7): xxxv

During the early years of the twentieth century the *Wisconsin Medical Journal* carried advertisements for buggies and automobiles, as well as physicians' driving coats.

petition among practitioners. Specialists, public health officers, visiting nurses, and even hospital ambulances from nearby cities now directly competed with the country practitioner. Patients also started motoring to specialized physicians located in neighboring urban centers. All of this resulted in the decline of individual rural practice.[97]

Wisconsin physicians increasingly turned to specialized practices. General practitioners with forty or more years of practice living in communities of fewer than 2,000 people earned the lowest physician incomes in 1930. Such physicians reported a gross income of $2,773 per year, $1,486 after expenses. These figures are in marked contrast with the earnings of specialists practicing in Milwaukee County for the same number of years. Their reported gross income was $21,560 per year, $8,814 after expenses.[98]

The Great Depression cast further economic gloom on the fortunes of many practitioners and changed the medical environment. A Madison physician, Chester Kurtz, wrote a fictionalized essay in 1930, identifying the factors necessary for success in medical practice.[99] Kurtz posited a hypothetical situation in which a Dr. McWilliams was recommended to a new resident of a small city of 4,000 people as the best of seven general practitioners. Four factors made McWilliams successful. He kept abreast of the modern developments in medical science, he was thorough in his work, he owned an adequately equipped medical office, and he had good business sense.

McWilliams not only kept up with the medical literature, he also spent his summers studying at nearby medical schools. He kept complete patient histories and consulted with specialists whenever appropriate. His office laboratory made routine blood and urine tests, as well as more sophisticated examinations. McWilliams had a small fluoroscope, a basal metabolism apparatus, a diathermy machine, and a lamp for ultraviolet treatments. He kept accurate account records and billed his patients promptly. McWilliams also participated in community affairs, involving himself in local politics, serving as a member of the local board of health, and assisting in financial drives, including one for the construction of a new hospital. Some public speaking and church work rounded out the model physician.[100] Kurtz's creation vividly captures the contemporary values and ideals shared by a majority of American physicians.

An exercise in nostalgia? A final, gallant attempt to save the fading generalist? Perhaps. In 1930 medical practice was adjusting to newer standards of efficiency. Expensive medical education was becoming a "capital investment," office practice was plagued by the burdens of "overhead," and the traditional spirit of medical altruism seemed threatened.[101] Yet the future of medicine was bright, concluded one Wisconsin physician. Life had been prolonged nearly eleven years since 1915, Cornelius A. Harper declared in 1930, and he anticipated that if "the medical profession had an opportunity to apply the modern principles of scientific medicine that life could be prolonged from at least seven to ten years" more.[102] Although the new century had brought new problems, it had also brought progress and a hope for better times to come.

Notes

1 W. H. Washburn, "Medical Practice in Wisconsin," *Wisconsin Medical Journal* 20 (1921–22): 324.

2 For a review of the prevalent diseases in mid-nineteenth century Wisconsin, see J. V. Stevens, "Getting Down to Cases," *Wisconsin Magazine of History* 20 (1936–37): 390–403.

3 J. Mitchell, President's Address, *Proceedings of the Wisconsin State Medical Society* (Janesville: C. Holt, 1857), p. 14.

4 Ibid., p. 32.

5 For an overview, see E. H. Ackerknecht, "Diseases in the Middle West," in *Essays in the History of Medicine* (in honor of David J. Davis, M.D., Ph.D.) (Chicago: University of Illinois Press, 1965), pp. 168–81. For the impact on a single county, see W. S. Middleton, "Cholera Epidemics in Iowa County, Wisconsin," *Wisconsin Medical Journal* 37 (1938): 1–7.

6 For a summary of mid-nineteenth-century American medical education, consult William Frederick Norwood, *Medical Education in the United States before the Civil War* (Philadelphia: University of Pennsylvania Press, 1944).

7 One of the notable exceptions was Joseph Hobbins (1816–1894), a pioneer Madison surgeon who systematically percussed and auscultated Camp Randall inmates applying for service-connected disabilities (Joseph Hobbins Papers, State Historical Society of Wisconsin, Madison, Wis.).

8 G. W. Jenkins, "Reminiscences of Some Earlier Medical Practice in Wisconsin," *Wisconsin Medical Journal* 8 (1909–10): 551.

9 Horace B. Willard, "Diary Recording Events of Dr. Willard's Medical Practice in Aztalan and Watertown 1856–58," Horace B. Willard Papers, 1849–1858, State Historical Society of Wisconsin, Madison, Wis.

10 See fee bill adopted by the Western Medical Society of Wisconsin and issued December 1849, Department of the History of Medicine, University of Wisconsin–Madison.

11 Dr. Tom O. Edwards made the presentation; *Proceedings* (1857), p. 36.

12 P. T. Harstad, ed., "A Civil War Medical Examiner: The report of Dr. Horace O. Crane," *Wisconsin Magazine of History* 48 (1964–65): 227.

13 Jenkins, "Reminiscences," p. 552.

14 See various accounts such as Jessica Rowley, "The Rowley Family of Doc-

tors" (1952), and Fred W. Riehl, "Brief Reminiscences of Medicine Fifty Years Ago" (1938), State Historical Society of Wisconsin. A sketch of William H. Oviatt (1839–1899), written by Gertrude Gessler, appeared in the *Clintonville* (Wisconsin) *Tribune Gazette* on August 18, 1965.

15 J. V. Stevens, "The Pioneer Wisconsin Family Physician," *Wisconsin Magazine of History* 17 (1933–34): 389.

16 One physician, Simon Miller (1848–1935), of Mondovi, Wisconsin, mentions using such a burner. See his daughter's account in the *Mondovi Herald*, Friday, May 3, 1935, p. 1.

17 Rowley, "The Rowley Family."

18 Centennial anniversary section: "William Herriman Fox, M.D.," *Wisconsin Medical Journal* 40 (1941): 629. Some of Fox's papers are in the State Historical Society of Wisconsin, Madison, Wis.

19 J. C. Reeve, "A Physician in Pioneer Wisconsin," *Wisconsin Magazine of History* 3 (1919–20): 308.

20 Fee bill, Western Medical Society of Wisconsin, December 1849, Department of the History of Medicine, University of Wisconsin–Madison.

21 This fee bill was donated by A. J. Wiesender to the State Historical Society of Wisconsin, Madison, Wis. See announcement in the *Wisconsin Medical Journal* 57 (1958): 506.

22 Marcus Bossard, *Eighty-One Years of Living* (Minneapolis: Midwest Printing Co., 1946), pp. 33–34.

23 L. G. Sorden, *Lumberjack Lingo* (Spring Green: Wisconsin House, 1969). For further information see J. P. Cox, "General Practice in Northern Wisconsin," *Wisconsin Medical Journal* 3 (1904–5): 643–47.

24 Fred C. Burke, "Recollections of Early Day Medical Practice in a Sawmill Village," Fred C. Burke Papers, State Historical Society of Wisconsin, Madison, Wis.

25 See Chapter 5 in this volume.

26 The four cases had occurred between October 1868 and February 1870. See report by Dr. Mason in *Transactions of the Wisconsin State Medical Society* 4 (1870): 12–16. Hereafter the title *Transactions* stands for both *Transactions of the Wisconsin State Medical Society* (1867–1879) and *Transactions of the State Medical Society of Wisconsin* (1880–1902).

27 John Favill, "On the Relations the Profession Holds and Ought to Hold towards Community," *Transactions* 6 (1872): 25–28.

28 N. Senn, "Necrosis and Its Treatment," ibid., pp. 33–51.

29 L. G. Armstrong, "Recent Improvements in Surgery," *Transactions* 8 (1874): 38–42.

30 J. Bull, "The First Experimental Surgical Laboratory in Milwaukee," *Marquette Medical Review* 32 (1966): 17–18. For some details on Senn, see the personal notes of one student, G. J. Kaumheimer, "Recollections of a Pioneer Milwaukee Physician," *Milwaukee Medical Times*, April 1931, pp. 17–21.

31 N. Senn, "Recent Progress in Surgery," *Transactions* 15 (1881): 76–119.

32 For details of the discussion see *Transactions* 15 (1881): 22–25.

33 A general discussion of antiseptic surgery was transcribed in *Transactions* 19 (1885): 23–32.
34 E. W. Bartlett, "Fraternally Yours," Presidential Address, ibid., p. 153.
35 J. S. Walbridge, "Report on Practice," *Transactions* 17 (1883): 31.
36 N. Senn, "Recent Progress in Surgery," *Transactions* 15 (1881): 82.
37 Jenkins, "Reminiscences," p. 554.
38 C. M. Gould, "Rational Therapeutics," *Transactions* 21 (1887): 172–76.
39 N. M. Dodson, "New Remedies," *Transactions* 17 (1883): 93.
40 J. G. Meachem, Jr., "Report on New Remedies," *Transactions* 15 (1881): 154.
41 F. H. Day, "New Remedies," *Transactions* 12 (1878): 119–20.
42 Ibid., p. 123.
43 See "Address by Governor Peck," *Transactions* 25 (1891): 6.
44 L. W. Beebe, "Reminiscences of a Northern Wisconsin Doctor," *Wisconsin Medical Journal* 40 (1941): 146.
45 See Judith Walzer Leavitt, "Public Health in Milwaukee, 1867–1910" (Ph.D. diss., University of Chicago, 1975), p. 95.
46 W. F. Whyte, "The Treatment of Laryngeal Diphtheria by Antitoxin," *Transactions* 3 (1897): 363–68.
47 J. F. Pember, "Serotherapy; with Special Reference to the Reduction of the Mortality Percentage since the Use of Diphtheria Antitoxin," *Transactions* 35 (1901): 131–54.
48 W. B. Metcalf, "Widal's Reaction in Typhoid Fever," *Transactions* 31 (1897): 321–31. See also manuscript materials on Janesville, Wisconsin, edited by J. V. Stevens, State Historical Society of Wisconsin, Madison, Wis.
49 J. E. Habbe, "Milwaukee's Radiologic Heritage," *Wisconsin Medical Journal* 64 (1965): 125–29.
50 J. S. Janssen, "My Early Experiences with the X-Ray," *Milwaukee Medical Times* 9 (August 1936): 16, 41–43.
51 S. H. Friend, "Clinical Report of Cancer of Breast under Treatment by the X-Ray," *Transactions* 36 (1902): 115–16.
52 "Address by Governor Peck," *Transactions* 25 (1891): 5.
53 R. St. Lawrence Noble, "Recollections," in papers from Waukesha County Medical Society, Wisconsin State Medical Society Women's Auxiliary Papers, 1836–1946, State Historical Society of Wisconsin, Madison, Wis.
54 William Osler, *Modern Medicine, Its Theory and Practice*, 7 vols., (Philadelphia: Lea Bros., 1907) "Introduction," 1:xxxiii.
55 B. C. Brett, "Presidential Address," *Transactions* 28 (1894): 36–46.
56 G. D. Ladd, "Aseptic Surgery," *Transactions* (1895): 69–79.
57 Ibid., p. 71.
58 S. M. B. Smith, "Reminiscences of a Family Doctor," sketch of medical practice and hospitals in the Wausau area dated August 20, 1953, State Historical Society of Wisconsin, Madison, Wis.
59 W. E. Ground, "In Memory of John Baird, M.D., 1860–1942," *Wisconsin Medical Journal* 42 (1943): 524.

60 F. W. Epley, "President's Address," *Transactions* 30 (1896): 52.

61 T. C. Malone, "The General Practitioner and the Surgeon," *Transactions* 32 (1890): 123.

62 E. C. Helms, "The Passing of the Family Physician," ibid., p. 238.

63 W. T. Sarles, "The Medical Practitioner," *Transactions* 34 (1900): 60–67.

64 C. R. Bardeen, "Hospitals in Wisconsin," *Medical Blue Book of Wisconsin 1925* (Milwaukee: State Medical Society of Wisconsin, 1925), p. 256. The article is reprinted in *Wisconsin Medical Journal* 24 (1925): 49–51, XXVI–XXX (June); XXIV–XXVI (July); XXVI–XXVIII (August); 222–224, 275–81, 284, XXVI–XXVIII (October).

65 Bossard, *Eighty-One Years*, p. 65.

66 R. St. Lawrence Noble, "Recollections."

67 Editorial comment: "The Telephone and the Doctor's Fee," *Wisconsin Medical Journal* 5 (1906–7): 187.

68 H. B. Favill, "The Avoidance of Malpractice Litigation," *Transactions* 26 (1892): 374–83.

69 B. T. Phillips, "President's Address," *Transactions* 27 (1893): 34–41.

70 H. Reineking, "President's Address," *Transactions* 33 (1899): 58.

71 Editorial comment: "The Question of Protective Insurance," *Wisconsin Medical Journal* 6 (1907–8): 166.

72 Letter by Armin Mueller, "The Physician as Accuser," ibid., p. 239.

73 Society Proceedings: "Medical Defense," ibid., pp. 493–96.

74 Editorial comment: "Medical Defense," ibid., pp. 480–81.

75 J. M. Dodd, "The Annual Address of the President of the State Medical Society of Wisconsin," *Wisconsin Medical Journal* 11 (1912–13): 1–4.

76 W. E. Ground, "The Ideal in Medicine," *Wisconsin Medical Journal* 7 (1908–9): 59–67.

77 T. J. Redelings, "Annual Address of the President of the State Medical Society of Wisconsin," *Wisconsin Medical Journal* 14 (1915–16): 181–86.

78 Editorial: "Your Duty!" *Wisconsin Medical Journal* 15 (1916–17): 482.

79 G. Windesheim, "Annual Address of the President of the State Medical Society of Wisconsin," *Wisconsin Medical Journal* 17 (1918–19): 173.

80 J. S. Evans, "Cardiac Disturbances from the Standpoint of Military Service," ibid., pp. 213–18.

81 Editorial: "Venereal Diseases and Peace," ibid., p. 412.

82 Editorial: "Group Medicine," ibid., pp. 336–37.

83 Washburn, "Medical Practice," p. 326. See also G. S. Custer, "The Development of Group Practice in the Midwest and Wisconsin," *Wisconsin Medical Journal* 75, No. 7 (July 1976): 32–37.

84 "Six Physicians Founded Marshfield Clinic Fifty-Nine Years Ago," *Marshfield News Herald*, June 24, 1975, p. 5.

85 "Biographical Sketches of Wisconsin Physicians," Wisconsin State Medical Society Women's Auxiliary Papers, 1836–1946, State Historical Society of Wisconsin, Madison, Wis.

86 See A. S. Jackson, "Conclusions Based on a Study of Four Thousand Cases of Goitre," *Annals of Surgery* 79 (1924): 840–44.

87 C. R. Bardeen, "Address of the President," *Wisconsin Medical Journal* 19 (1920–21): 209–16.
88 "Survey of Group Clinics," Minutes of the House of Delegates, *Journal of the American Medical Association* 80 (1923): 1932. A decade later the AMA denounced a recommendation by the Committee on the Costs of Medical Care calling for group practice.
89 H. P. Greeley, "The Use of Precise Methods in Medicine," *Wisconsin Medical Journal* 17 (1918–19): 131–35.
90 For an assessment of contemporary methods, consult John A. Kolmer and Fred Boerner, *Laboratory Diagnostic Methods* (New York: Appleton, 1925).
91 See Logan Clendening, *Modern Methods of Treatment* (St. Louis: C. V. Mosby, 1924), esp. pp. 159–70.
92 M. P. Earles, "Salvarsan and the Concept of Chemotherapy," *Pharmaceutical Journal*, April 18, 1970, pp. 400–402.
93 Personal communication from Dr. Marvin G. Peterson, Lake Mills, Wis.
94 Bardeen, "Hospitals in Wisconsin," pp. 235–67.
95 M. L. Berger, "The Influence of the Automobile on Rural Health Care, 1900–29," *Journal of the History of Medicine* 28 (1973): 319–35.
96 Ibid., p. 321.
97 O. B. Fiedler, "County Lacks Facilities," *Wisconsin Medical Journal* 22 (1923–24): 495.
98 *Progress Report of Special Committee on Distribution of Medical Services in Wisconsin* (Madison: State Medical Society of Wisconsin, 1932).
99 C. M. Kurtz, "How One General Practitioner Increased His Usefulness and Bettered His Position in the Community," *Wisconsin Medical Journal* 29 (1930): 354–56.
100 Ibid., pp. 360–62.
101 Editorials: "Scientific Medicine," *Wisconsin Medical Journal* 29 (1930): 20–21, and "The Responsibility for Leadership," ibid., pp. 278–79.
102 C. A. Harper, "The Future of Medicine," the President's page, *Wisconsin Medical Journal* 29 (1930): 642–43.

Elizabeth Barnaby Keeney,
Susan Eyrich Lederer, and Edmond P. Minihan

Sectarians and Scientists:
Alternatives to Orthodox Medicine

Since territorial days, Wisconsin's regular physicians have competed with a host of unorthodox practitioners representing a broad spectrum of the healing arts. At one end were out-and-out quacks, eager to make a fast dollar at the expense of the sick and gullible. At the other were the so-called sectarians, many of whom possessed M.D. or equivalent degrees, but who sincerely disagreed with regular physicians over the best therapy. This chapter focuses primarily on the latter group: the homeopaths, hydropaths, and eclectics, who flourished in the nineteenth century, and the osteopaths and chiropractors, who achieved prominence during the twentieth. It also discusses the rise of a unique method of religious healing, Christian Science, which first gained popularity in Wisconsin near the turn of the century.

Sectarian appeal during the early years of statehood rested largely on the inadequacies of regular medicine — or allopathy, as it was commonly called. Although the age of "heroic" therapy, famous for its massive bleedings and purgings, was waning by mid-century, public suspicion of regular practice remained high, creating an atmosphere conducive to alternative forms of healing. At times irregular physicians represented one-third of all practitioners in Wisconsin,[1] a condition that forced allopaths to contend for public support with homeopaths, hydropaths, herb-using eclectics, and various self-styled doctors. An anonymous poet, writing in a Milwaukee newspaper, depicted the situation in 1868:

> Allo shouts with lungs stentoric, "lance and mortar to the fray,"
> Homeo, with a laugh sardonic, orders Allo's hosts away;
> And commands that "powder pellets on the adversary play"—
> Hydropath and Herbatarius stand aside and smile to see
> How their prospects look the brighter, as those doctors disagree.[2]

Of Allo's three chief competitors, Homeo achieved by far the greatest popularity in nineteenth-century Wisconsin. Developed by a German physician, Samuel Hahnemann (1775–1843), homeopathy became famous for its twin principles of drug action: that a drug that produces a given symptom in a healthy person will alleviate that symptom in an ill person (the law of similars); and that drug potency increases as dosage decreases. By 1825 this system of medicine had reached America, where it spread rapidly through the Northeast and Midwest. The warm response given it on this side of the Atlantic stemmed in part from the contrast between homeopathic and allopathic therapy; to many Americans, harmless, infinitesimal doses of drugs producing no harsh effects seemed eminently preferable to the excessive bleeding and violent medication associated with regular medicine.[3]

Homeopathy came to Wisconsin in 1846, when two practitioners arrived in Milwaukee from the East. One of them left within a year, but the arrival of James S. Douglas from New York a short time later more than made up for the loss. Douglas, destined to become one of the city's most distinguished sectarians, almost immediately began publishing a small weekly magazine, the *Homeopathic Medical Reporter*. Not long thereafter he founded a homeopathic medical society and opened a homeopathic pharmacy. The pharmacy sold medical books and supplies as well as drugs, which Douglas and his associates compounded and triturated on the premises.[4]

The ambitious Dr. Douglas soon found himself at odds with local allopaths, who apparently resented his success and his eagerness to win converts. When, under Douglas's influence, a former president of the Milwaukee City Medical Association adopted homeopathy in 1848, the association expelled the apostate physician for sacrificing "truth and substance" as well as "conscience, honor, dignity and delicacy."[5] Like most regular medical societies, the Milwaukee City Medical Association prohibited members from having social or professional relationships with sectarian physicians.[6] "It was perfectly understood," explained the *Homeopathic Medical Reporter*, "that the members [of the association] were not only to avoid recognizing us as physicians, but that they were not to know us as human beings in any of the relations of life."[7] Reports of harassment, both verbal and physical, were not uncommon.[8] According to one story, a regular of the "extremely heroic variety" nearly precipitated a duel by attacking a homeopath with "a complete inundation of tobacco juice flavored with brandy, square in the face and eyes."[9]

At times homeopaths took the offensive. When cholera threatened Milwaukee in 1866, for example, Douglas touched off a front-page debate in local newspapers by contrasting the allegedly rational and effective homeopathic treatment for cholera with the deadly allopathic therapy. Regular physicians responded in kind, and the debate raged on for three months.[10] Such outbursts, however, like expulsions and physical attacks, became less frequent as the century progressed. Many homeopaths and allopaths learned to live together in peace, remaining on friendly terms despite the obvious potential for conflict.[11]

Although homeopathy failed to displace regular medicine from its dominant position in the state, homeopaths did remarkably well for themselves. By the early 1870s, when homeopaths accounted for only 5.9 percent of all physicians in the United States (according to an American Medical Association survey), they constituted 14.9 percent of practitioners in Wisconsin — the highest by far for any state in the union.[12] In Milwaukee, with its large German population, new homeopaths arrived nearly every year, swelling the homeopathic community at times to a third of the city's medical population. But even in Milwaukee, many homeopathic physicians and patients were non-German.[13] Cities like Janesville, Beloit, Madison, and Eau Claire — none of which attracted large numbers of Germans — all supported thriving homeopathic practices, with homeopaths reportedly controlling 75 percent of all medical practice in Eau Claire during the 1860s.[14]

In 1874, approximately a quarter century after the arrival of the first homeopath, 183 known homeopaths were practicing in 44 different counties, located largely in the populous southern and central regions of the state. Milwaukee remained the leading homeopathic center with 16 practitioners, followed by Kenosha with 6, and Oshkosh and Fond du Lac with 5 each. Only 70 of the 183 homeopaths (38 percent) reported graduating from medical school, the most popular institutions being the nearby Hahnemann Medical College in Chicago, with 26 alumni, and the Cleveland Homeopathic Hospital College, with 18 alumni. Of the remaining medical school graduates, the majority had received regular degrees before switching to homeopathy.[15] Five of the state's homeopaths were women.[16] At least one of them, Dr. Julia Ford of Milwaukee, specialized in treating women and children.[17]

S. J. MARTIN, M. D.,

HOMŒOPATHIC

Physician and Surgeon,

RACINE, WISCONSIN.

———•———

OFFICE and RESIDENCE 1st and 2d Door North M. E. Church, Main Street.

Office Hours, 8 to 9 A. M., 1 to 3 and 6 to 7 o'clock P. M.

HOMŒOPATHIC MEDICINES.

A large supply constantly on hand.   Family cases furnished and re-filled.

Allen & Cory's Racine City Directory for the Years 1872–73, p. 200
(State Historical Society of Wisconsin)

During the 1870s, when Dr. S. J. Martin practiced homeopathy in Racine, Wisconsin had a higher percentage of homeopaths than any state in the nation.

Those homeopaths without medical degrees had often learned the rudiments of medicine from an older physician and then simply set up practice on their own. A Door County homeopath, Dr. David Graham, described his entry into the profession as follows:

I studied medicine and practiced nearly two years under an old allopathic physician in the state of Ohio, in 1844 and 1845, but before I had an opportunity to graduate I became disgusted with the treatment and abandoned practice entirely. I became acquainted about that time with Dr. Ross, who was practicing homeopathy in the village of Painesville, Lake county, Ohio. I told him my difficulties and obtained a small case of medicines and a small book of instructions and came to Wisconsin. I studied my little book and prescribed the little pills in my own family until 1852, when I obtained Jahr's "Manual of Homeopathic Practice," with medicines, and began to prescribe for my neighbors, and was soon given the title of Dr. Graham.[18]

By means of manuals and kits like those used by Dr. Graham, the influence of homeopathy spread far beyond the practice of individual homeopaths to the farthest reaches of the state. Do-it-yourself guides at first served primarily in the absence of homeopathic physicians, later as a supplement to professional care. Among the widely circulated local works were Douglas's *Practical Homeopathy for the People* and Lewis Sherman's *Therapeutics and Materia Medica for the Use of Families and Physicians*, both written and published in Milwaukee.[19] These manuals often accompanied family medical kits, which contained the most commonly used homeopathic medicines.[20]

The citizens of Wisconsin demonstrated their appreciation of various homeopaths by electing or appointing them to prestigious civic and institutional offices. Homeopaths won appointments as physicians to the state prisons and schools, as city physicians, as health commissioners. Some also served on the staffs of predominantly regular hospitals, like St. Mary's Eye and Ear Infirmary in Milwaukee. In 1871 Madisonians elected Dr. James Bowen, a homeopath, mayor of the state capital.[21]

Like regular physicians, homeopaths published their own professional journals, established their own medical schools (though not in Wisconsin), and organized their own medical societies.[22] After several abortive attempts the state's homeopaths finally, in 1865, created a viable state medical society, the Homeopathic Medical Society of the State of Wisconsin.[23] After twelve years of existence it claimed a membership of 90, although only about two-thirds of these attended the annual meetings.[24] At such meetings members presented clinical and scientific papers, conducted society business, discussed impending legislation, and reevaluated their relationship with allopaths. The topics of medical ethics and etiquette occupied hours of discussion, which sometimes resulted in disciplinary action against members for using secret formulas, displaying bogus diplomas, or espousing another sect. The yearly meetings also provided an opportunity for socializing and usually featured an extravagant banquet. Drugs might be fine in small doses, but certainly not food![25]

Wisconsin homeopaths also supported one of the country's earliest societies for medical research: the Milwaukee Academy of Medicine (not to be confused with the later regular society of the same name). At a time when medical research received little more than lip service, a group of Milwaukee homeopaths devoted considerable time and energy to scientific experimentation. As an academy member, Douglas frequently tested homeopathic remedies on himself to prove them by the law of similars, and he collaborated with his protégé Lewis Sherman in standardizing drugs sold at their pharmacy. But the height of homeopathic experimentation in Wisconsin came in 1878, when the academy sought to test the efficacy of high dilutions. Using double-blind techniques long before they became popular, experimenters distributed placebos and medicines to healthy subjects and cooperating physicians

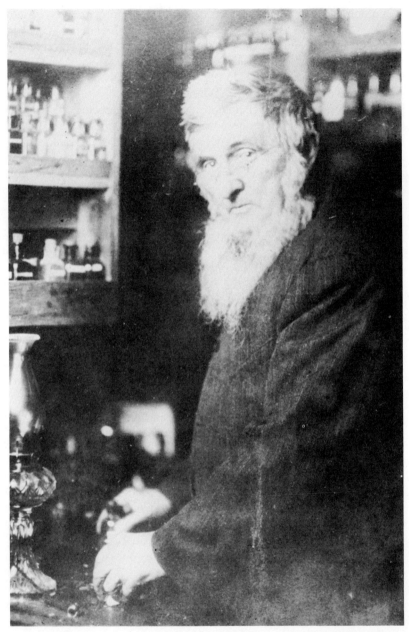

Courtesy of Arthur Brickbauer, Plymouth, Wisconsin
(Department of the History of Medicine, University of Wisconsin–Madison)

Dr. George Brickbauer, a homeopathic physician, in his Elkhart Lake office.

The results, however, can best be described as inconclusive.[26]

Eclectic physicians, the second largest group of sectarians in both Wisconsin and the nation during the second half of the nineteenth century, provided another alternative to regular medicine. Founded in the late 1820s by Dr. Wooster Beach, a regular medical school graduate from New York, the eclectic system purported to embrace the best of all therapies, regular or irregular. In practice, eclectics simply replaced the lancet and mineral drugs used by allopaths with an assortment of botanic preparations. Like allopaths and homeopaths, they valued medical education and practiced surgery and obstetrics as well as medicine.[27] Although homeopaths slightly outnumbered them nationally, eclectics built great strength in a midwestern belt running through Ohio, Indiana, Illinois, and Missouri, where they clearly outdistanced their homeopathic rivals and captured nearly 10 percent of the medical practice.[28]

The first eclectics arrived in Wisconsin in the 1840s to an apparently warm reception. As one pioneer wrote in 1850: "There is no state in the Union (except Ohio perhaps), where reform takes so well as here, for I doubt not that there are five hundred places where a Reformer eclectic might make a good living if no more. Therefore, if you have a surplus of practitioners and desire for them locations, send them to our State—There is room—'the harvest is plenty but the laborers are few.'"[29] Despite such prospects, eclectics failed to accomplish in Wisconsin what they achieved in other midwestern states. In 1871 only 5.6 percent (52) of the state's physicians identified themselves as eclectics, compared with 14.9 percent (138) for homeopaths and 67.6 percent (626) for allopaths.[30]

Unlike homeopathy, which thrived in the cities, the eclectic approach did best in the small towns and rural areas of the state, where botanical medicine had deep roots.[31] Most members of the Wisconsin State Eclectic Medical Society, organized in 1870, resided in places like Eau Claire, La Crosse, Baraboo, and Wausau. Few eclectics practiced in Milwaukee or Madison, although Milwaukee had the dubious honor of being the home of Wisconsin's only eclectic medical school: the Wisconsin Eclectic Medical College. This ephemeral institution opened in 1894 and graduated its first and only class in 1896.[32] Apparently it was little more than a degree mill—and an embarrassment to respectable eclectics. When the school shut down and Chicago authorities arrested its dean "for selling diplomas and for misusing the United States mails," the state eclectic medical society expressed only relief.[33]

By this time the eclectics, unable to keep pace with the rapid advances of scientific medicine and to attract and retain good young physicians, were beginning to fade both nationally and locally. A survey of state eclectic medical societies in 1894 noted that Wisconsin's "old members are staunch, straightforward, good men, but the younger ones, however emulous of their place and honors, seem hardly their equals in Eclectic enthusiasm and energy."[34] Clearly the sect could not prosper long under such conditions.

In contrast to the homeopaths, with their infinitesimal doses, and the eclectics, with their botanic preparations, hydropathic physicians, who formed Wisconsin's third major sect, treated their patients with water. Developed by Vincenz Priessnitz, a Silesian farmer, hydropathy began attracting American followers in the 1840s and flourished until the 1860s. To cure the sick, American hydropaths utilized a multitude of baths, compresses, and douches, often in combination with exercises and special diets. Although much hydropathy was self-administered, hydropathic physicians were available at so-called water cures, which offered facilities for treating and accommodating patients. At no time, however, did the number of professional hydropaths exceed a few hundred nationally and a handful in the state.[35]

Wisconsin supported major water cures at Kenosha and Madison, with smaller establishments at Berlin, Janesville, Kilbourn City, Palmyra, and Sheboygan.[36] The state's most attractive water cure, if not its

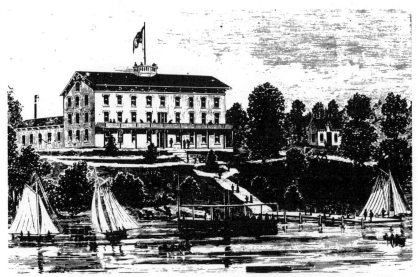

Madison: Past and Present, 1852–1902
(Madison: Wisconsin State Journal, n.d.), p. 101

Madison's beautiful Lake Side Water-Cure, built as a hydropathic institution in 1855, became a popular resort after the Civil War.

most successful, opened in Madison in 1855. Known variously as the Madison Water-Cure, the Lake Side Water-Cure, and the Lake-Side Retreat, this establishment, with accommodations for over one hundred patients, occupied a scenic tract on the south side of Lake Monona with a view of the capitol. There was, reported a local newspaper, "not a more beautifully situated water-cure in the American Union."[37]

Despite its geographical advantages and repeated efforts to make it "the model cure of the West," the institution apparently did not flourish. Within three years, five resident physicians came and left, and a sixth, Dr. S. M. Landis of Philadelphia, remained a few years at most.[38] The hydropaths, it seems, did not get along well with the town's regular practitioners, and on one occasion an argument between a water-cure doctor and a prominent allopath over the merits of drug therapy nearly turned into a fight on the mayor's lawn.[39] Although several of his predecessors had mixed hydropathy with more traditional therapeutics, Landis professed to treat all diseases "on *strictly* Hygienic and Physiological principles." For $8 to $12 a week, patients could enjoy the benefits of "the ELECTRO-CHEMICAL BATH [obviously the house specialty], Russian Vapor, Dry Vapor, and Air Baths, the Movement Cure, and a variety of curative adjuncts." Clothes for lake bathing rented for $1.[40]

In 1862 Dr. Russell T. Trall, one of the founders of the American hydropathic movement and owner of a large water cure in New York City, announced his imminent purchase of the Madison establishment and invited "the bilious and horribly drugged invalids of the Western country" to come for treatment. Although he intended to make Madison the western headquarters of the water-cure movement, his plans never materialized. When he and the owners failed to agree on a fair price, the water cure became a resort.[41]

Advertisements for hydropathic physicians, placed by several Wisconsin towns in the 1850s, suggest that demand exceeded supply.[42] Perhaps because of this shortage, domestic practice of hydropathy was widespread. The *Water-Cure Journal*, published in New York, carried numerous accounts from Wisconsin of successful home cures for such complaints as burns, fevers, scarlatina, whooping cough, and rheumatism. Wisconsin readers also frequently solicited free medical advice from the editors. Sometimes the domestic practitioners followed up home treatment with a visit to one of the state's water cures.[43]

Although the water-cure movement barely survived the Civil War, Kenosha boasted two *homeopathic* water cures in the 1870s, and remnants of that practice could be found in Wisconsin as late as the early twentieth century.[44] Stimulated by the writings of a German priest, Sebastian Kneipp, hydropathy staged a comeback in the 1890s, and we know of at least one Kneipp sanitarium operating in La Crosse in the early 1900s.[45] Of greater importance, however, was the opening in 1903 of a branch of the famous Battle Creek Sanitarium, run by Dr. John Harvey Kellogg, inventor of corn flakes and other health foods. Kellogg, a graduate of both hydropathic and regular medical schools, had been directing a Seventh-day Adventist water cure in Battle Creek, Michigan, since 1876. In 1881 the Adventist prophetess, Ellen G. White, visited Madison and expressed interest in establishing a branch of the Battle Creek institution in Wisconsin, but the death of her husband a short time later led to a postponement in plans. It was the turn of the century before Adventists finally opened hydropathic treatment rooms and a vegetarian restaurant in the city. The success of these ventures encouraged them to purchase the old Madison Water-Cure property on Lake Monona and to build a new 40-bed structure, the Madison Sanitarium, dedicated in 1903.[46]

Unlike Madison's previous hydropaths, the Adventists flourished. After their first year in operation they reported a net gain of $9,000 — despite performing more than $6,000 in charity work.[47] Staffed by a husband-wife medical team and nurses from its own Missionary Nurses' Training School, the Madison Sanitarium offered a range of services, including obstetrics and surgery. Not wishing to appear sectarian, the sanitarium emphasized its nonexclusive approach to therapy: "Electrotherapy, Massotherapy, Hydrotherapy, Allopathy, Surgery, Diet and exercise are the measures resorted to in the treatment of disease in this place." Nevertheless, the sanitarium specialized in hydrotherapy and included morning and afternoon water treatments in its weekly rates. Patients suffering from stomach disorders wore "moist girdles" at night.[48] The sanitarium survived into the 1930s.

In addition to its allopaths, homeopaths, eclectics, and hydropaths, Wisconsin in the early 1870s provided employment for over one hundred assorted other practitioners, who constituted 11.6 percent of the state's practitioners.[49] Unlike many of the sectarians we have discussed, these doctors presumably had little or no formal training; some may have been quacks, who remained legally free to practice medicine in the state. Reputable physicians from the three major schools — allopathy, homeopathy, and eclecticism — grew increasingly concerned about such unqualified persons, as well as about incompetents within their own ranks.[50] The Homeopathic Medical Society of the State of Wisconsin, for example, refused membership to a graduate of the Hahnemann Medical College in St. Louis because the school was neither respectable nor rigorous.[51] But such actions, being extralegal, had only symbolic value.

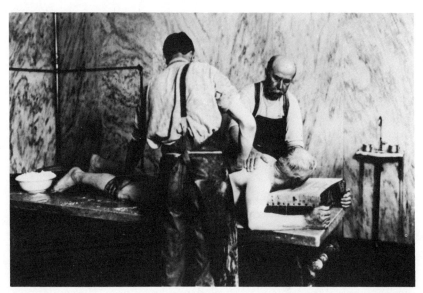

Courtesy of the Lewis W. Hine Collection,
George Eastman House, Rochester, N.Y.

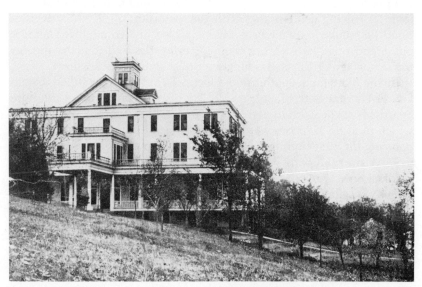

State Historical Society of Wisconsin, WHi(X3)32549

The Madison Sanitarium, a branch of Dr. John Harvey Kellogg's world-famous Battle Creek Sanitarium, opened in 1903. It featured water treatments like that being administered above.

During the last quarter of the century representatives of all three schools began agitating for the passage of restrictive legislation that would prevent unqualified persons from practicing in the state. Only a few decades earlier, allopaths would have been happy to see homeopaths and eclectics denied the right to practice medicine, but now regulars allied themselves with these sectarians in order to control the *real* quacks. After nearly twenty years of collective effort—and not a little mutual distrust—the three schools succeeded in 1897 in obtaining the creation of a state board of medical examiners, composed of three allopaths, two homeopaths, and two eclectics, with five votes needed to approve a license.[52]

By this time, however, the eclectic movement had already crested, and the homeopaths, though numerically at their peak, were showing signs of decreased vitality. After winning their most important victory, they found themselves in the paradoxical position of losing the war for survival. During the first two decades of the twentieth century, they lost ground rapidly, partially from their inability to maintain high-quality medical schools and partially from defections. "Homeopathy is losing out through the laziness of its doctors through[out] the state," declared a Fort Atkinson homeopath in 1912. "It is easier for us to follow the prescriptions of other schools than to get down and study out our own."[53] Having collaborated with the sectarians on licensing legislation, the regular state medical society in 1903 invited qualified homeopaths and eclectics to break their sectarian ties and join the regular physicians under the common banner of scientific medicine.[54]

By the 1930s homeopathic and eclectic strength had dwindled to such low levels that both schools feared loss of representation on the state board of medical examiners.[55] The inevitable occurred in 1953, by which time the eclectics were too feeble even to protest and the aging homeopaths were finding it difficult to locate members "physically able to serve on the board."[56] The last few meetings of the Homeopathic Medical Society of the State of Wisconsin were a far cry from the gala events of the late nineteenth century; the final banquet consisted of sixteen members eating lunch at a coffee shop.[57] Deprived of a place on the examining board, the homeopaths reluctantly admitted defeat. "With the passage of the new law," wrote one survivor,"the incentive for further existence [of the state society] has been removed."[58] But even facing the end, some homeopaths dreamed of a miracle. In the minutes of what turned out to be the society's last meeting, in 1953, the secretary noted poignantly: "This society remains an active one."[59]

As the nineteenth-century sects gave way to scientific medicine, new alternative systems of healing—of varying importance—arose to take their place. Naturopathy, which sought healing through diet and hygiene, neither attracted many adherents nor won legal recognition in the state. Christian Science, which taught healing by right thinking, remained essentially a health-oriented religion. Osteopathy and chiropractic, however, evolved into full-blown medical sects, which specialized in treating illness by manual manipulation of the skeletal system, especially the spine. Indigenous to the Midwest, both systems reflected the needs of rural populations, who had little patience for arcane Latin phrases and long-term therapies.[60] Without invoking invisible germs or hospitalizing their patients, osteopaths and chiropractors often provided quick relief for problems like lower back pain, to which regular physicians were inattentive and for which regular medicine was inefficacious. Moreover, osteopaths and chiropractors, who initially shunned drugs and major surgery, charged lower fees than regular physicians.

At a time when women saw few professional opportunities, Christian Science, osteopathy, and chiropractic offered them careers in the healing arts. Early in the twentieth century, women accounted for over 90 percent of Christian Science practitioners in Wisconsin, for 30 percent of the osteopaths, and for approximately 20 percent of chiropractors.[61] As the *Wisconsin Osteopath* noted in 1898, osteopathy not only furnished women "lucrative employment," but catered to their needs as patients.[62] Because osteopaths did not require the removal of clothing for either treatment or examination, they saved women the embarrassment of undressing in front of strangers. The same was true of chiropractors and Christian Scientists.

These twentieth-century sectarians, however, faced barriers unknown to the early homeopaths, eclectics, and hydropaths, who started practicing when the only requirements were a saddlebag full of medicines and self-confidence. The days of unregulated practice ended in 1897 with the creation of the state board of medical examiners, which required aspiring physicians either to present a diploma from a reputable medical school or to pass an examination in medicine and surgery. The new sectarians, who had no representation on the original board, thus confronted the problem of how to treat patients without violating the law. Christian Scientists, osteopaths, and chiropractors each solved the dilemma in a different way: Christian Scientists with a court ruling that their healing activities did not constitute the practice of medicine, osteopaths with an appointment to the state board of examiners, and chiropractors with the creation of a separate licensing board.

Of the three, Christian Scientists arrived in Wisconsin first, gaining a solid foothold in the state by the 1880s.[63] (The first Christian Science church in America was built in Oconto in 1886[64]). Founded by Mary

Baker Eddy, a New England mystic who had once practiced homeopathy, Christian Science disavowed traditional medicine and denied
the very existence of sickness, disease, and death.[65] Practitioners,
trained by the church in metaphysical healing, used verbal persuasion
to rid patients of their false beliefs (i.e., symptoms of illness), or employed silent prayer, supposed to be efficacious over long distances.

Wisconsin's first Christian Science practitioners, two graduates of
Eddy's Massachusetts Metaphysical College named Silas and Jennie
Sawyer, began healing in Milwaukee in 1883. The following year they
offered instruction in Christian Science healing, a major attraction of
the church during its early years. Before long Christian Science "dispensaries" (present-day reading rooms) appeared, offering spiritual and
moral healing as well as physical treatment of disease. By the early
twentieth century, Christian Science practitioners could be found in
nearly every corner of the state, although the greatest concentration
lived in Milwaukee.[66] At least some of these practitioners maintained
busy practices; one Milwaukee woman claimed to have treated 670 persons in four years, generally charging only a modest fee for her services.[67]

Such activities, apparently in violation of the medical practice act of
1897, did not go unchallenged for long. In May 1900, Mrs. Crecentia
Arries and Miss Emma Nichols, two Christian Science practitioners
from Milwaukee, went on trial for practicing medicine without a license.[68] Other states had already prosecuted Christian Scientists on similar charges, but the church welcomed the opportunity to vindicate and
clarify the status of its practitioners. The outcome of the trial hinged on
the question of whether Christian Scientists were practicing medicine
or religion. The prosecution maintained that they were practicing medicine, pointing out that Mrs. Eddy's text, *Science and Health*, described
Christian Science surgery, Christian Science anatomy, and Christian
Science obstetrics. The defense attorney replied that Christian Science
practitioners should not be regulated by the medical practice act because they never administered drugs, never performed surgery, never
manipulated the body or even touched their patients. The medical
practice act discriminated against Christian Scientists, he argued, because it allowed them neither to receive a medical license (without
studying scientific medicine) nor to be represented on the examining
board. Unpersuaded, the judge found the defendants guilty of practicing medicine without a license. On appeal the women won acquittal in
a higher court, a decision that cleared the way for Christian Scientists
in Wisconsin to heal without fear of the law.

Orthodox physicians, who had fought for a quarter-century to eliminate just such practices, were less than happy with the reversal. Ralph

Elmergreen, a Milwaukee physician, denounced the higher court's decision as a "crime, originating in hysteria and perversion, and grafted on the principles of the denial of matter and the irresponsibility of man. A learned judge, listening to the ravings emanating from the sepulchral voice of an ephemeral fifteenth century delusion — for Eddyism is but a rescrudescence of this mediaeval mania. A great judge tolerating these monumental farces!"[69]

Although most physicians would not have expressed themselves so strongly, many seemed genuinely concerned for a number of reasons. First, Christian Scientists, who generally charged little for their services and drew their clients from the middle and upper classes, who were able to pay the fees of regular physicians, hurt the medical profession economically. Second, the sect's refusal to accept medical treatment led to reports of "Christian Science suicide" and stories about the children of Christian Scientists dying needlessly.[70] Third, the group's disavowal of public health laws, such as those requiring the reporting of communicable diseases, threatened the health of the community. As the editors of the *Milwaukee Medical Journal* remarked: "The well-known disbelief of this cult in the contagiousness of communicable diseases is a direct menace to society."[71] The eventual vindication of Arries and Nichols, however, left regular physicians with few weapons besides verbal protests.

Osteopaths, who appeared in Wisconsin a decade after the first Christian Science healers, practiced a system of medicine devised by Andrew Taylor Still (1828–1917).[72] The son of a Methodist missionary-physician in the American West, Still studied medicine with his father and briefly attended the College of Physicians and Surgeons in Kansas City. Although he did not obtain a medical degree, he practiced allopathic medicine for a number of years, until drug therapy failed to save the lives of three of his children, who died of spinal meningitis. Disillusioned, Still formulated a new theory of disease, based on a mechanical view of the human body. At the core of his system was his belief that "the brain of man was God's drug-store and had in it all liquids, drugs, lubricating oils, opiates, acids, and anti-acids, and every quality of drugs that the wisdom of God thought necessary for human happiness and health."[73] When misalignment of the skeleton interrupted the natural flow of the body's fluids through the nervous and arterial systems, sickness occurred. To effect a cure, one needed only to restore the correct anatomical relationship by manipulating the musculoskeletal structure, thus allowing "God's drug-store" to do its work. "An intelligent head will soon learn," taught Still, "that a soft hand and a gentle move is the hand and head that get the desired results."[74] Following the opening of the first osteopathic school in Kirksville, Missouri, in 1892, osteopathy spread rapidly through the Midwest, becoming especially popular in Still's home state of Missouri and in neighboring Iowa.

The first evidence of osteopathy in Wisconsin appears in 1893, when Still's son, Charles, accepted an invitation to practice in Diamond Bluff, on the Mississippi.[75] Although the townspeople guaranteed 25 patients, young Still remained only a month. Four years passed before osteopaths settled permanently in the state, in the Milwaukee area. These pioneers, nearly all graduates of the Northern Institute of Osteopathy in Minneapolis, included a husband-wife team, Essie and Leslie Cherry, who wasted no time in founding their own school.

One of twelve osteopathic schools in the nation, the Cherry's Milwaukee Institute (later College) of Osteopathy opened its doors in 1898. Its two-year curriculum, spread over four five-month terms, combined the study of such traditional subjects as anatomy, physiology, and chemistry with osteopathic diagnosis, osteopathic jurisprudence, and clinical practice of osteopathy.[76] (The institute maintained a clinic, which treated patients for $2.50 a visit or $25.00 a month.) There was no instruction in materia medica or major surgery. The institute's faculty consisted of three D.O.'s (doctors or diplomates of osteopathy), one "professor" (the former physical education director of the local Y.M.C.A.), and an M.D. who had graduated from Rush Medical College and served on the Chicago Board of Health. The school survived only three years, graduating 25 students, before rising educational standards forced it out of business.

By 1900, when the sect encountered its first legal challenge, 19 osteopaths, located primarily in Milwaukee, Racine, and Janesville, were practicing in the state. In September of that year the Milwaukee district attorney's office, at the behest of two members of the state board of medical examiners, swore out a warrant for the arrest of Swen A. L. Thompson, D.O., who had been practicing in the city for about a year.[77] The warrant charged Thompson with violation of the medical practice act, a misdemeanor, because he called himself a physician but possessed neither a license from the state nor a diploma from a recognized medical college.

The state's osteopaths, who had been expecting prosecution, welcomed this opportunity to determine their legal status. Like the Christian Scientists, they contended that the practice of osteopathy did not constitute the practice of medicine because it did not involve the prescription of drugs or the performance of surgery. Warren B. Davis, secretary-treasurer of the Milwaukee College of Osteopathy, pointed out that "when the legislature passed the law referred to [in 1897], there

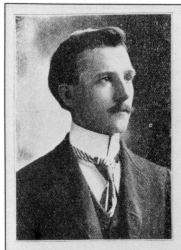

Osteopathy - -

Is a Science,

which recognizes causes heretofore overlooked by the medical fraternity. The Osteopathic physician on account of his thorough training in anatomy, locates causes of disease unknown to the other methods of treatment. This is why Osteopathy cures where other methods fail.

Office consultation is FREE, and investigation is solicited. Home treatment only by special arrangement. The treatment is never too severe, but always adapted to the strength of the patient.

A. U. JORRIS, D. O.,

(Member of the A. A. A. O. and Vice President of the W. S. O. A.)
Formerly on staff of operators at the Northern Institute of Osteopathy. Now at

LA CROSSE, WISCONSIN.

Write for booklet explaining Osteopathy.   **3d Floor McMillan Building.**

The Wisconsin Osteopath 2 (1900): 125

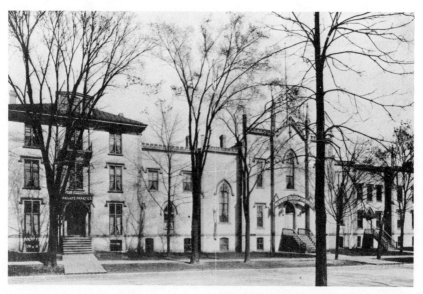

The Wisconsin Osteopath 2 (1900): advertising supplement

The first osteopaths came to Wisconsin in the 1890s. The Milwaukee College of Osteopathy, opened in 1898, lasted for only three years.

were no osteopaths in the state, and we firmly believe that it was not the intention to cover the practice of osteopathy, but to cover the giving of drugs and the use of the knife for cure of disease."[78] Davis also compared the medical education of allopaths and osteopaths, noting that "our course compares favorably to theirs, with this important exception — where they teach materia medica, we teach osteopathy . . . the drug doctors cannot be honestly against us on account of our lack of knowledge of the human body."[79] Despite such arguments, the court found Thompson guilty and fined him $50.

Stung by this decision, the osteopaths in 1901 asked the legislature to create a separate licensing board for osteopathy, recognizing it as a healing art distinct from the practice of medicine. But regular physicians, denouncing the proposed bill as "only a scheme for practicing medicine by a short cut," successfully blocked its passage.[80] They did agree, however, to a compromise measure providing for the addition of one osteopath to the three allopaths, two homeopaths, and two eclectics already on the state board of medical examiners. Since five votes were still required to approve a license, such an arrangement would, the regulars believed, keep the number of licensed osteopaths to a minimum. As the secretary of the State Medical Society of Wisconsin observed: "The requirements are so high it is safe to say that but few, if any, osteopaths will ever be able to meet them, or, if they do, they are bound to be pretty good men."[81] Endorsed by both osteopaths and allopaths, the compromise bill passed the legislature, making Wisconsin the first state to allow osteopathic representation on its medical examining board and the sixteenth to recognize osteopathy legally.[82] To the surprise of the regulars, osteopaths experienced little difficulty obtaining licenses under the new system.

Despite their new legal standing, osteopaths remained an object of suspicion among regulars. In an attack on sectarians, quacks, and smut, Ralph Elmergreen, the outspoken chairman of the medico-legal section of the state medical society, denounced "Hahnemanian inanities, Eclectic absurdities, Osteopathic asininities, and Christian Science insanities."[83] The editors of the *Milwaukee Medical Journal*, who regretted that osteopaths had been recognized at all, called them "the most irregular of irregulars."[84] Nevertheless, as the century progressed, these early animosities faded, partially, it seems, because osteopaths increasingly adopted the ways of regular medicine and because they never became as popular in Wisconsin as elsewhere in the Midwest. In 1930 there were only 3 osteopaths per 100,000 population in Wisconsin, compared with 6 in Minnesota, 7 in Illinois, 14 in Iowa, and 17 in Missouri (see Table 3.1).[85]

Table 3.1. Sectarian Practitioners in Midwestern States and in the United States, 1930

Location	Osteopaths		Chiropractors		Christian Scientists	
	Number	Per 100,000 of population	Number	Per 100,000 of population	Number	Per 100,000 of population
Wisconsin	89	3	600	20	202	7
Illinois	551	7	645	8	881	12
Iowa	358	14	834	34	129	5
Minnesota	157	6	374	15	162	4
United States	7,644	6	15,989	13	8,848	7

Source: Louis S. Reed, *The Healing Cults: A Study Of Sectarian Medical Practice: Its Extent, Causes, and Control* (Chicago: University of Chicago Press, 1932), pp. 131–34.

Early in the twentieth century a number of osteopaths began combining a modest amount of drugs and surgery with manipulation. They were known as mixers. Purists, led by the elder Still, opposed this trend, but the movement toward mixed practice continued. In 1915 Wisconsin osteopaths won the legal right to perform surgery, and by the 1930s upgraded osteopathic colleges were routinely teaching materia medica and pharmacology.[86] Consequently, it became increasingly difficult for the public to distinguish osteopathic physicians from regular ones. Although osteopaths continued to experience difficulty obtaining hospital privileges, they had little trouble gaining admission into the State Medical Society of Wisconsin. But like the homeopaths and eclectics before them, they soon discovered that acceptance came with a price: the more they practiced like orthodox physicians, the less they could claim to be an alternative to regular medicine.

The last, and perhaps most successful, of the major sects to come to Wisconsin was chiropractic. As the story goes, Daniel David Palmer (1845–1913), an Iowa grocer and magnetic healer, accidentally discovered the secret of chiropractic in 1895 when he restored the hearing of a janitor by manually adjusting the man's spine.[87] From this and other experiences, Palmer concluded that all disease resulted from misalignments, called subluxations, of the vertebrae, which obstructed the flow of nervous force. Therapy consisted of returning the affected vertebrae to their normal positions.

Not surprisingly, many people initially confused chiropractic with osteopathy. In 1914 the *Journal of the American Medical Association* identified chiropractic as

a freak offshoot from osteopathy. Its followers assert that disease is caused by pressure on the spinal nerves and can be eradicated by "adjusting" the vertebrae. It is the sheerest kind of quackery, practiced largely by men whose general knowledge is as limited as their knowledge of anatomy, and who are profoundly ignorant of the fundamental sciences on which the treatment of disease in the human body depends.[88]

Neither chiropractors nor osteopaths appreciated this confusion. Osteopaths looked upon Palmer and his followers as "fakeopaths" who had stolen many of their ideas from Still, while chiropractors insisted that "Chiropractic is no more Osteopathy than a dead dog is Osteopathy."[89]

Shortly after the founding in 1897 of the Palmer Institute and Chiropractic Infirmary in Davenport, Iowa, chiropractors moved into other midwestern states — with the sheriff often one step behind. Palmer himself spent six months in jail in 1903 for practicing without a license, and over the next few decades chiropractic cases, estimated at 15,000, clogged the nation's courtrooms.[90] Like the early osteopaths, chiropractors argued that because they did not practice medicine, they should not be subject to the medical practice laws.

The chiropractic penetration of Wisconsin began about 1906, when two chiropractors, E. J. Whipple and G. W. Johnson, were arrested in La Crosse for practicing *osteopathy* without a license.[91] The night before their trial the pair skipped town and headed across the river to Minnesota, from whence they could not be extradited for a misdemeanor. They soon turned up, however, nearly destitute, in Wabasha, Wisconsin, billing themselves as the "famous La Crosse Chiropractors." Arrested by the sheriff and returned to La Crosse, Whipple and Johnson found themselves confined to the little-used second floor of the La Crosse jail. During an exercise period one cold morning they managed to get locked out of their cell, clad only in light night clothes. When the jailer discovered them hours later, they were running up and down the hallway trying to keep warm, their lips blue from the cold. Their ultimate fate remains unknown, although the state board of medical examiners may have had them in mind when it reported in 1906 the conviction of "incompetent and disreputable men" in La Crosse for violating the medical practice act.[92] Certainly the escapades of Whipple and Johnson, covered gleefully by local newspapers, scarcely contributed to the good name of chiropractors in Wisconsin.[93]

The arrival in La Crosse of a Japanese chiropractor in January 1907 returned chiropractic to the front pages. Reportedly sent by Palmer to test the Wisconsin law and aware of the recent difficulties of Whipple and Johnson, Shegataro Morikubo immediately retained counsel "in case of trouble."[94] Little is known about Morikubo except that he impressed the newspapers with his scholarly credentials, claiming, in addition to his degree in chiropractic, a Ph.D. (of undetermined origin and field) and membership in the Tokyo Academy of Science. He seems to have enjoyed the limelight and confidently urged La Crosse residents to "Come and See You Doubting Thomas."[95]

Trouble came as anticipated. Arrested in the summer, Morikubo went to trial in August on charges of illegally practicing osteopathy. Represented by the prominent firm of Morris and Hartwell (Morris was then a state senator), Morikubo put up a vigorous defense. Charles Linning, an expert witness for the defense who held degrees from two chiropractic colleges, explained the difference between chiropractic and osteopathy: chiropractors used only spinal manipulation whereas osteopaths employed a variety of therapeutic techniques. Either D. D. Palmer or his son B. J. (the record is unclear) also testified in Morikubo's behalf. The prosecutor countered with a woman osteopath who had attended the Palmer College of Chiropractic under an assumed name. She told the court of having heard rumors that Morikubo had come to Wisconsin specifically to test the licensing law. The jury was unimpressed. After deliberating 25 minutes, it found the learned Dr. Morikubo not guilty of practicing osteopathy.[96]

Disappointed, the chairman of the state board of medical examiners threatened to prosecute Morikubo on a second charge, of practicing the art of healing and receiving money for that activity. Senator Morris, however, talked him out of it, arguing that it might be seen merely as Japanese persecution, a national issue at the time. The chairman agreed to look for another chiropractor to prosecute—if one could be found in the state. How long it took him to find one we do not know, although there is evidence from the early 1910s that chiropractors were still being arrested for practicing osteopathy without a license.[97] In 1915 the chiropractors won a minor victory when the legislature passed a law allowing them to practice their art, provided that they prominently displayed signs reading "Not Registered or Licensed in Wisconsin."[98] Clearly Wisconsin chiropractors had made an early commitment to court and chamber as the principal arenas for establishing their legitimacy.

In 1925 the chiropractors, who maintained a powerful lobby in Madison, used their political skills to win legislative approval for the creation of a separate chiropractic licensing board, independent of the one that licensed regulars and other sectarians. Fourteen states had already passed chiropractic acts of one kind or another by 1920, and during the next decade twenty-five more states did so.[99] The Wisconsin chiropractic act established an examining board, the members to be appointed by the governor from a list of names submitted by the Wisconsin Chiropractic Association (founded in 1911, incorporated in 1948). Although the regular state board of medical examiners continued to monitor the activities of chiropractors, this arrangement gave chiropractors a licensing autonomy unavailable to any other sect. They secured such favorable legislation partly because the efforts of regular physicians remained uncoordinated and ineffective in thwarting chiropractic.[100]

Wisconsin's chiropractors did not, however, win all they wanted. They could not use the title "doctor" (until 1975), and they had to meet certain standards required of all healers in the state. The same legislature that gave chiropractors a separate examining board simultaneously passed a basic-science act, the first in the nation, requiring that all applicants for licenses to treat the sick, regardless of sect, must pass an examination in anatomy, physiology, chemistry, bacteriology, and diagnosis. Although the bill contained a clause exempting those already practicing in the state, chiropractors saw it as a sinister attempt to "exterminate" them.[101] Ironically, its effect was just the opposite; the basic-science requirement ultimately raised the standards, and thus prestige, of chiropractic.

Five years after the creation of the chiropractic examining board, 600 chiropractors — 20 for every 100,000 residents — were practicing in Wisconsin, compared with 202 Christian Science practitioners and only 89 osteopaths. In the upper Mississippi valley, only Palmer's home state of Iowa, with 34 chiropractors per 100,000 population, had a higher ratio (see Table 3.1).[102] Chiropractic strength in Wisconsin dropped below five hundred in the 1940s, but rose again to nearly six hundred in the early 1970s.[103] Generally, chiropractors did best in the northern and western parts of the state, especially in the rural areas, and worst in urban centers like Milwaukee. Both regular physicians and chiropractors, however, tended to avoid the rural northern regions of the state.

Like the osteopaths before them, chiropractors split into two factions: the "straights," who relied almost exclusively on adjustment and who controlled the Wisconsin Chiropractic Association (WCA), and the "mixers," who incorporated diet, vitamins, and other therapies into their practice and who in 1955 created a second organization, the Society of Wisconsin Chiropractors (SWC).[104] Among the leaders of the SWC was a Kenosha chiropractor, Robert L. Grayson, whose efforts to adopt new techniques brought him into conflict with the law. A search of his office turned up an incriminating array of diagnostic and therapeutic devices: a Plasmatic machine (to increase body heat), a syringe for administering DeWells Detoxicolon Therapy (a mineral enema), a vibrating Raylax table, a Mayofasciatron low-voltage generator, an ultraviolet lamp, a Heartometer (to measure vascular tone and strength of heart beat), Vitameter and Oster massagers, an X-ray machine, a Micro-Dynameter (to diagnose subluxations and other conditions), and an "electrosonic" instrument. On the basis of such evidence, the state supreme court in 1958 found Grayson guilty of using methods beyond those legally defined as chiropractic.[105]

Perhaps in retaliation for suspected WCA involvement in the Grayson affair, the SWC charged a prominent WCA member, L. S. Toftness of Cumberland, with using a machine called a Neurolinometer, or "black box." The WCA-controlled chiropractic examining board refused to take action against Toftness on the grounds that his device was only a research model used for diagnostic purposes, but the SWC nevertheless succeeded in embarrassing its rivals. In 1961, at the request of the SWC, Glenn Koehler of the University of Wisconsin College of Engineering examined the "black box" and found it to be a simple amplifier, incapable of performing any useful diagnostic function.[106]

By 1970 the two quarreling societies had resolved their differences and merged into one organization, retaining the name of the dominant Wisconsin Chiropractic Association. Reunited, the chiropractors quickly scored a series of impressive legal victories: the right to receive insurance payments under workmen's compensation, Medicare, and Medicaid, the privilege of using the title "doctor," and the inclusion of a chiropractic option in health-insurance policies. In the years since Morikubo's arrest in La Crosse, they had learned their political lessons well.

They had also learned how to attract large numbers of patients, particularly among farmers, retired people, self-employed workers, and individuals without higher education. During a 1978 survey of public attitudes toward chiropractic in the state, over a third of the respondents reported having consulted a chiropractor, often for a back problem. An overwhelming majority expressed satisfaction with the care they had received — and with the fees they had paid — although an even higher percentage liked the medical care (if not the bills) they had received from regular physicians. Surprisingly, in view of the medical profession's continued hostility toward chiropractic, 4 percent of the chiropractic patients stated that they had been referred by a medical doctor.[107] Clearly, the sectarian spirit remained alive and well in Wisconsin.

Notes

1 J. M. Toner, "Tabulated Statistics of the Medical Profession of the United States," *Transactions of the American Medical Association* 22 (1871): 155–56.

2 Milwaukee *Sentinel*, June 2, 1866, p. 1.

3 William G. Rothstein, *American Physicians in the Nineteenth Century: From Sects to Science* (Baltimore: Johns Hopkins University Press, 1972), pp. 237–39.

4   [J. S. Douglas], "History of Homeopathy in Milwaukee," *Homeopathic Expositor* 1, no. 7 (1867): 1–8; [Uranus] Wingate, "Medical History of Milwaukee, 1841–1851," manuscript, Medical History Room, Milwaukee Academy of Medicine; and advertising material in the Kremers Reference Files, School of Pharmacy, University of Wisconsin–Madison.

5   Minutes, Milwaukee City Medical Association, March 3, 1848, April 7, 1848, May 18, 1848, June 1, 1848, and July 27, 1848, Milwaukee Academy of Medicine.

6   "Rules of Etiquette," Milwaukee City Medical Association, 1845, Milwaukee Academy of Medicine.

7   Thomas Lindsley Bradford, "Homeopathy in Wisconsin," in *History of Homeopathy and Its Institutions in America*, ed. William Harvey King, 4 vols. (New York: Lewis Publishing Co., 1905), 1:337–38.

8   See for example *Homeopathic Expositor* 1 (1867), nos. 7, 8, 10.

9   W. W. Day, "The Rise and Progress of Homeopathy in Eau Claire, Wis.," *Homeopathic Expositor* 1, no. 10 (1867): 5.

10 Milwaukee *Sentinel*, May 15, 1866; May 17, 1866; May 19, 1866; May 22, 1866; May 23, 1866; June 6, 1866; and June 12, 1866.

11 Day, "Rise and Progress of Homeopathy," pp. 4–6.

12 Toner, "Tabulated Statistics," pp. 155–56. Rhode Island had the second highest percentage of homeopaths, with 12.8 percent; Michigan was third, with 11.0 percent. Among Wisconsin's other neighbors, Minnesota had 8.6 percent, Iowa had 5.9 percent, and Illinois had 6.3 percent.

13 Eunice B. Bardell, "The Role of German Immigrants in the Health of Early Settlers of Milwaukee," *Acta Congresus Internationalis Historiae Pharmacia* (Bremae, 1975), pp. 179–89.

14 Day, "Rise and Progress of Homeopathy," pp. 4–6; [Douglas], "History," pp. 1–8; "The Origin of Homeopathy in Madison, Wisconsin and Vicinity," *Homeoepathic Expositor* 1, no. 10 (1867): 6–7.

15 Lewis Sherman, *Directory of the Homeopathic Physicians in the State of Wisconsin* (Milwaukee: Lewis Sherman, 1874), pp. 2–24.

16 Ibid., pp. 2–9.

17 Minutes of the Homeopathic Medical Society of the State of Wisconsin, 1872–1890, State Historical Society of Wisconsin, Madison, Wis. Hereafter cited as HMSSW Minutes.

18 Quoted in Bradford, "Homeopathy in Wisconsin," p. 341.

19 James S. Douglas, *Practical Homeopathy for the People, Adapted to the Comprehension of the Non-Professional and for Reference by the Young Practitioner* (Milwaukee: by the Author, 1866); and Lewis Sherman, *Therapeutics and Materia Medica for the Use of Families and Physicians* (Milwaukee: Cramer, Aikens & Cramer, 1878).

20 Advertising material in the Kremers Reference Files, School of Pharmacy, University of Wisconsin–Madison.

21 E. Cleave, *Cleave's Biographical Cyclopedia of Homeopathic Physicians and Surgeons* (Philadelphia: Galaxy Publishing Co., 1873), pp. 124, 296–97; "Origin of Homeopathy," pp. 6–7; Judith Walzer Leavitt, "Public

Health in Milwaukee, 1867–1910" (Ph.D. diss., University of Chicago, 1975), p. 51; Milwaukee *Sentinel*, April 1, 1877, p. 4; and Marianne Herriott, "Placards and Pretenders: The Dane County Medical Society in the 'Good Old Days,'" *Wisconsin Medical Journal* 75, no. 10 (October 1976): 16.

22 Homeopathic journals published in Wisconsin include *The Homoeopathic Expositor* (Milwaukee, publication started in 1866), *Madison Homoeopathist* (Madison, 1854), *Wisconsin Medical Record* (Milwaukee, 1855), and *Milwaukee Homeopathic Medical Reporter* (Milwaukee, 1848). No extant copies of the *Madison Homoeopathist* and *Wisconsin Medical Record* are known.

23 HMSSW Minutes, October 18, 1865.

24 *Constitution, By-Laws and History of the Homeopathic Medical Society of the State of Wisconsin* (Milwaukee: Burdick & Armitage, 1877), pp. 8–9.

25 HMSSW Minutes, June 13, 1878; June 11, 1879; June 1, 1881; May 29, 1894; and "The Homeopathic Medical Society of Wisconsin Banquet, Thirty-Eighth Annual Convention, Plankinton House Milwaukee, May Twenty-First, Nineteen Hundred and Two," in Pamphlet Collection, State Historical Society of Wisconsin, Madison, Wis.

26 Helen Sherman to Edward Kremers, August 2, 1901, Kremers Reference Files, School of Pharmacy, University of Wisconsin–Madison; Samuel O. L. Potter and Lewis Sherman, *Papers on the Milwaukee Test of the Thirtieth Dilution* (Milwaukee: Milwaukee Academy of Medicine, 1878); and artifact in the Kremers Reference Files labeled "A Test of the Thirtieth-Dilution, Therapeutic."

27 Rothstein, *American Physicians*, p. 226; Ronald L. Numbers, "The Making of an Eclectic Physician: Joseph M. McElhinney and the Eclectic Medical Institute of Cincinnati," *Bulletin of the History of Medicine* 47 (1973): 155–66; Louis Frederick Frank, *The Medical History of Milwaukee, 1834–1914* (Milwaukee: Germania Publishing Co., 1915), p. 106.

28 Toner, "Tabulated Statistics," pp. 155–56.

29 *Eclectic Medical Journal* 11 (1850): 384.

30 Toner, "Tabulated Statistics," pp. 155–56.

31 Rothstein, *American Physicians*, p. 228.

32 Alexander Wilder, *History of Medicine* (New Sharon, Maine: New England Eclectic Publishing Co., 1901), p. 743.

33 "One Fake College Gone," *Eclectic Medical Journal* 57 (1897): 244.

34 Alexander Wilder, "Eclectic State Societies," *Eclectic Medical Journal* 54 (1894): 175–76.

35 Harry B. Weiss and Howard R. Kemble, *The Great American Water-Cure Craze: A History of Hydropathy in the United States* (Trenton: Past Times Press, 1967).

36 Milwaukee *Sentinel*, April 26, 1877, p. 2; November 19, 1873, p. 3; January 3, 1873, p. 2; November 27, 1876, p. 2; and *Water-Cure Journal* 22 (1856): 88.

37 *Wisconsin State Journal*, April 24, 1855, p. 2. We wish to thank Janet S. Numbers for information on the Madison Water-Cure.

38 Weiss and Kemble, *Great American Water-Cure Craze*, pp. 222–23. Weiss and Kemble identify only five of the physicians; a sixth appears in the *Water-Cure Journal* 21 (1856): 108. The same journal (26 [1858]: 28) also mentions a seventh hydropath who may have joined the Madison Water-Cure.

39 E. A. Kitteredge, "Wisconsin—Its Climate, &c.," *Water-Cure Journal* 22 (1856): 36.

40 "Lakeside Retreat," *Water-Cure Journal* 25 (1858): 46.

41 R. T. Trall, "Rambling Reminiscences—No. 6: Our Trip to the West," *Water-Cure Journal* 33 (1862): 27; "Madison Water-Cure," ibid., p. 83.

42 *Water-Cure Journal* 16 (1853): 135; 13 (1852): 128; and 20 (1855): 89.

43 *Water-Cure Journal* 16 (1853): 103–4.

44 Sherman, *Directory*, pp. 18, 21.

45 The *La Crosse Argus* for June 30, 1906, carried an advertisement for a Kneipp and Nature Cure Sanitarium.

46 C. P. Farnsworth, "The Madison (Wis.) Sanitarium," *Advent Review and Sabbath Herald* 82 (1905): 19–20.

47 Ibid., p. 20.

48 Ibid.; *The Madison Sanitarium* (Madison, 1903), pp. 29, 31; "Madison's Sanitarium," in *Madison, Past and Present* (Madison: Wisconsin State Journal, 1902), p. 199.

49 Toner, "Tabulated Statistics," pp. 155–56.

50 See Chapter 4 in this volume.

51 HMSSW Minutes, June 1, 1879.

52 See Chapter 4 in this volume.

53 "Lazy Doctors Causing Decline, Says Dr. Nair," *Milwaukee Sentinel*, May 30, 1912.

54 See Chapter 4 in this volume.

55 HMSSW Minutes, May 23, 1930; June 2, 1932; and June 2, 1933.

56 Frederic E. Kosanke, Secretary of the Homeopathic Medical Society of the State of Wisconsin, to the American Institute of Homeopathy, 1953, in Kosanke Papers, State Historical Society of Wisconsin, Madison, Wis.

57 HMSSW Minutes, May 19, 1946, and May 18, 1952; Frederick E. Kosanke to A. H. Ferguson, undated letter, in Kosanke Papers, State Historical Society of Wisconsin, Madison, Wis.

58 Kosanke to The American Institute of Homeopathy.

59 HMSSW Minutes, May 24, 1953.

60 Thomas McCorkle, "Chiropractic: A Deviant Theory of Disease and Treatment in Contemporary Western Culture," *Human Organization* 20 (1961): 20–22.

61 In 1905–6, the number of female Christian Science practitioners was 100 (91.8 percent of the total); *Christian Science Journal* 23 (1905–6): lxxiv–lxxv. In 1908, 15 of the 50 practicing osteopaths were women; Franklin Fiske, ed., *The Osteopathic Directory and A.O.A. Yearbook* (Kirksville, Missouri, 1908). In 1925, 119 of 593 chiropractors licensed were female; see Wisconsin State Board of Examiners in Chiropractic, Chiropractic Law, Rules and Regulations, September, 1925.

62 "Study Osteopathy," *Wisconsin Osteopath* 1 (1898): 14.

63 Kellogg Patton, "History of Christian Science in Wisconsin," typescript, 1938, State Historical Society of Wisconsin, Madison, Wis.

64 Robert Peel, *Mary Baker Eddy: The Years of Authority* (New York: Holt, Rinehart and Winston, 1977), p. 396.

65 For biographical information on Mary Baker Eddy, see Sydney E. Ahlstrom, "Mary Baker Eddy," in *Notable American Women 1607–1950*, ed. E. T. James and J. W. James, 3 vols. (Cambridge, Mass.: Harvard University Press, 1971), 1: 555–61.

66 Christian Science practitioners tended to be concentrated in urban areas; see Louis S. Reed, *The Healing Cults: A Study of Sectarian Medical Practice: Its Extent, Causes, and Control* (Chicago: University of Chicago Press, 1932), p. 73. In Wisconsin in 1905, 34 of 109 practitioners (31 percent) were located in Milwaukee, 10 were in Madison, and 6 were in Sheboygan; *Christian Science Journal* 23 (1905–6): lxxiv–lxxv.

67 A. C. Umbreit, ed., *Christian Science and the Practice of Medicine* (Milwaukee: Evening Wisconsin, 1900), p. 57.

68 Ibid. This is an exact transcript of the trial held in the police court of Milwaukee.

69 Ralph Elmergreen, "A Protest," *Milwaukee Medical Journal* 9 (1901): 205.

70 The *Reader's Guide to Periodical Literature* contains over 125 references to Christian Science in the years 1890–1910. For examples, see "Christian Science and Death Certificates," *Journal of the American Medical Association* 32 (1899): 1185; Edmund Andrews, "Christian Science: The New Theologico-Philosophic Therapeutics," ibid., p. 580.

71 "By Their Fruits Shall They Be Judged," *Milwaukee Medical Journal*, 19 (1911): 45.

72 Andrew Taylor Still, *The Autobiography of Andrew Taylor Still: With a History of the Discovery and Development of the Science of Osteopathy* (Kirksville, Missouri, 1897).

73 Ibid., p. 219.

74 Emmons Rutledge Booth, *The History of Osteopathy, and Twentieth-Century Medical Practice*, 2nd ed., rev. (Cincinnati: Jennings and Graham, 1905), p. 40.

75 Kirk W. Shipman, "Osteopathy in Wisconsin 1897–1940," typescript, 1940, State Historical Society of Wisconsin, Madison, Wis.

76 School bulletins and advertisements appeared in the *Wisconsin Osteopath*. Also see Booth, *History of Osteopathy*, p. 90.

77 "Dr. Thompson's Arrest," Milwaukee *Sentinel*, September 27, 1900.

78 "Test of Osteopathy," Milwaukee *Sentinel*, September 25, 1900.

79 Ibid.

80 *Milwaukee Medical Journal* 10 (1902): 110.

81 *Transactions of the State Medical Society of Wisconsin* 35 (1901): 20. Such a forecast proved erroneous, for in 1903 50 osteopaths practiced in the state; *Wisconsin Medical Journal* 2 (1903–4): 153.

82 Booth, *History of Osteopathy*, pp. 126–28.

83 Ralph Elmergreen, "Medical Mountebank," *Transactions of the State Medical Society of Wisconsin* 36 (1902): 189.

84 *Milwaukee Medical Journal* 9 (1901): 111.

85 Reed, *Healing Cults*, p. 131.

86 For a discussion of osteopathic education, see Bob E. Jones, *The Difference a D. O. Makes: Osteopathic Medicine in the Twentieth Century* (Oklahoma City: Times-Journal Publishing Co., 1978), pp. 19–29. See also Erwin A. Blackstone, "The AMA and the Osteopaths: A Study of the Power of Organized Medicine," *The DO* (1978): 1–20.

87 Russell W. Gibbons, *Chiropractic History: Lost, Strayed or Stolen* (Davenport, Iowa: Palmer College Student Council, 1976); and B. J. Palmer, *The Science of Chiropractic: Its Principles and Philosophies*, 3rd ed. (Davenport, Iowa: Palmer School of Chiropractic, 1917).

88 "Chiropractic," *Journal of the American Medical Association* 62 (1914): 1177.

89 Reed, *Healing Cults*, p. 38; *La Crosse Daily Chronicle*, July 2, 1907.

90 Reed, *Healing Cults*, p. 53.

91 La Crosse *Argus*, May 19, 1906.

92 *Wisconsin Board of Medical Examiners Reports*, December 31, 1906.

93 La Crosse *Argus*, June 16, 1906.

94 La Crosse *Daily Chronicle*, Jan. 29, 1907.

95 La Crosse *Daily Chronicle*, July 2, 1907.

96 La Crosse *Daily Chronicle*, August 15, 1907.

97 There were at least two other early prosecutions. The transcript of one, *State of Wisconsin* v. *S. R. Janeshecki*, was reprinted by the American Medical Association in 1911.

98 *Wisconsin Statutes*, 1915, Chap. 58, Sec. 1435e.

99 Thorp McClusky, *Your Health and Chiropractic* (New York: Milestone Books, 1957), p. 239. See John Harley Warner, "Organized Medicine's Opposition to Chiropractic: 1895–1970," manuscript, 1976, courtesy of the author.

100 See the correspondence of the Board of Examiners in Chiropractic for inquiries concerning individual chiropractors. See also the annual reports of the investigator of the state board of medical examiners for investigations into non-licensed or illegally practicing healers.

101 F. G. Lundy, *The Benfy Bill Analyzed* (Wisconsin Chiropractic Association, 1923), p. 1.

102 Reed, *Healing Cults*, pp. 131–34.

103 *Chiropractic Manpower, Wisconsin 1972* (report prepared by the Department of Health and Social Services, Division of Health), p. 1.

104 Articles of Incorporation, Society of Wisconsin Chiropractors, November 1, 1955 (Office of the Secretary of State, Madison, Wis.).

105 *State* v. *Grayson*, 5 Wis. (2nd) 203.

106 *Wisconsin State Journal*, June 9, 1961.

107 Daniel J. Duffy, *Public Attitude toward Chiropractic and Patient Satisfaction with Chiropractic in the State of Wisconsin* (privately published, 1978).

4 *Ronald L. Numbers*

Public Protection and Self-Interest:
Medical Societies in Wisconsin

The mid-nineteenth century was a terrible time for physicians, especially in sparsely settled areas such as Wisconsin. Transportation was poor, and medical journals appeared sporadically.[1] Many practitioners therefore lived in geographical and intellectual isolation. To make matters worse, they had to fight not only diseases, for which they were usually ill-equipped, but often their own colleagues. Dissension and discord were endemic in a profession already rent into competing sects. As we have seen in the previous chapter, in addition to the so-called regulars, or allopaths, who bled and purged, homeopaths prescribed their "little" pills, eclectics dosed with botanicals, and hydropaths promoted the water cure. Given this confusion and conflict, it is understandable that society took a rather disapproving view of the medical profession — and that regular physicians resented the indiscriminate public for giving "equal standing to the quack & the charlatan, to the Homeopathist & Hydropathist with the scientific & phylosophic physician."[2] In response to this deplorable situation, some farsighted regular physicians began advocating the creation of medical societies, long popular in the East, which would simultaneously elevate the profession and protect the public.[3]

On February 19, 1841, the Legislative Assembly of the Territory of Wisconsin passed a law permitting the incorporation of county and ter-

ritorial medical societies, reasoning that "well regulated medical societies have been found to contribute to the advancement and diffusion of
true science, and particularly of the healing art." The law required
county organizations to have at least five members and to be open to all
physicians and surgeons who possessed a diploma "from any incorporated medical college or society." A physician not possessing such a document could obtain one by examination, provided that "he shall have
arrived at the age of twenty-one years, has, at least, a good English education, and has studied medicine at least three years with some respectable practitioner, and can produce satisfactory evidence of good moral
character." Applicants who failed the examination or were unable to
meet the requirements still could practice medicine. The diploma was
purely symbolic. The law explicitly stated that none of its provisions
shall "be so construed as to prevent any person from practicing physic
and surgery within this territory, who is not a member of any of said
societies."[4]

The law also empowered Dr. M. C. Darling and twelve other physicians to meet in Madison in January 1842 to create the Medical Society
of the Territory of Wisconsin. This body was to be composed of delegates from the county societies, who served for the period of their elec-
tion, plus permanent members, only two of whom could be elected each
year from "among eminent physicians of this territory." Apparently the
incorporators hoped by this arrangement to create a prestigious association while at the same time preventing "the clogging of the Society with
too large a number."[5]

Such fears proved entirely unfounded. Only a few county societies
organized, and most of these chose not to send delegates to the territorial society.[6] In addition, only a handful of the elected permanent members bothered to attend the annual meetings, held in places like "a bor-
rowed barber's shop in the basement of the old United States Hotel, in
the village of Madison."[7] Undoubtedly the poor attendance was partially attributable to transportation difficulties, especially in winter,
when the meetings were scheduled. Dr. Harmon Van Dusen of Mineral
Point, a former president of the New York State Medical Society, reportedly spent two or three days traveling to the Milwaukee sessions.[8]
Few physicians were willing to sacrifice so much for so little, and even
the threat of expulsion for nonattendance did not help. By the early
1850s attendance was so low that two annual sessions were canceled for
lack of a quorum. No out-of-town physicians showed up in 1852 when
Van Dusen hosted the meeting in Mineral Point, and only three members turned up the next year in Janesville.[9]

To remedy this intolerable situation, the Wisconsin State Medical Society, as it was now called, in 1854 opened its ranks to any "regular physician in good standing." But even this drastic remedy did not save the organization. By 1856 a "profound lethargy" had set in, prompting the secretary to observe that "a want of professional pride seems to be the great desideratum with the medical profession in Wisconsin." A stranger wandering into one of the society's meetings might well think, he said, that only the host town was represented.[10] Throughout the late 1850s the society maintained only "a weakly existence," and "the few who attended were almost discouraged about its future." With the coming of war and the entry of many Wisconsin physicians into the army, the state medical society quietly faded away.[11]

After Appomattox "the surviving members of the Society, one by one, turned their thoughts to their honored association." Partly at the urging of former president Van Dusen, nine members met in Janesville on July 23, 1867, to reorganize the society.[12] By 1871 the association claimed 163 members, all but a dozen of whom had joined since the reorganization, and most of whom lived in the southern part of the state. Although the bulk of the membership came from small towns, Milwaukee had sixteen members; Madison, ten; Janesville, nine; and Fond du Lac, Mineral Point, and Racine each had five.[13] Over the next three decades the society nearly quadrupled, thanks in large part to the efforts of two indomitable secretaries, Dr. J. T. Reeve of Appleton, who served during the 1870s and 1880s, and Dr. C. S. Sheldon of Madison, whose tenure covered the next quarter-century. In the days before the existence of a paid staff and permanent headquarters, the secretary was all-important. He acted as chief recruiter, program director, editor, and exhorter, infusing a sometimes lethargic profession with what Sheldon called "Medical Society Spirit."[14]

The state medical society during the nineteenth century saw itself not only as the voice of the profession but also as the advocate of the people. Its purpose, as stated in the constitution, was fourfold: to promote the advancement of medical science, to cultivate a fraternal spirit among members of the medical profession, to conserve the public health, and to protect "ourselves and society" against the encroachment of "medical pretenders."[15]

In promoting medical science, the society in its early years often fell short of its ambitions. The annual sessions constituted the core of the society's activities, and the presentation and discussion of clinical cases took up much of the time. Each member not already on the program was expected to present at least one important case of his own. By sharing experiences in this way, the society hoped "the more successfully to combat diseases and accidents, in all their various forms and phases."[16]

Unfortunately, most of the required reports contributed little to science, and many merely provoked heated controversy. At one session a member described "a singular malformation" in a pig he had seen. Some exhibited new instruments or appliances. Occasionally the society attempted to diagnose patients actually brought to the meetings, but even the state's leading physicians were sometimes baffled. An examination of a woman suffering from a roaring in the right side of her head, for example, produced "a diversity of opinion . . . and no conclusion."[17]

When the society reorganized after the Civil War, it created standing committees on practical medicine, surgery, and obstetrics, which were to report each year on the "most practical improvements, discoveries, and advancements" in these fields. It also required each member "to give a complete and detailed written history of one case of disease occurring under his own observation comprising everything touching its etiology, pathology, symptomatology, nosology, diagnosis, prognosis, therapeutics and hygienics."[18] Although many papers continued to be of little value and a few "bordered on empiricism and considerable quackery," some were of great worth. "I approached the sick-bed of a person with puerperal fever with fear and trembling," testified one member, "until the discussions in this Society brought up certain things that led me out of it."[19]

A few members during the latter part of the century strove mightily to upgrade the society's scientific program. An outstanding example was Dr. Nicholas Senn of Milwaukee, considered by many to have been "the greatest surgeon, medical authority and writer the West had ever produced." He often experimented at night in an underground laboratory at home, and his innovative work in abdominal surgery won him international acclaim.[20] Senn joined the society in 1870 and served as its president in 1878–79, at the age of thirty-four. During the 1870s and early 1880s scarcely a year passed in which he did not give a paper or major report, always making sure to present the "practical" aspects of his work, which would be of greatest value to his audience.[21]

Time and again Senn defended scientific medicine against the less enlightened views of some of his colleagues. As late as 1881, when a Fond du Lac surgeon declared that it was not necessary "to go to all the trouble and nicety of carrying out Listerism in its fullness," Senn had to explain the *practical* advantages of antiseptic surgery:

It is true, we have to spend more time at the first dressing. A wound that you may dress, perhaps, in five minutes with ordinary slovenly method, you may consume an hour in dressing according to antiseptic principles, but it is your first and your last dressing. . . . the trouble which may be incurred during the first dressing should be no plea for an abandonment of the blessings of antiseptic surgery.[22]

Three years later he was justifying the germ theory to a skeptical colleague, who questioned Robert Koch's views on the bacillary origin of tuberculosis. "I believe," said Senn firmly, "if any one fact has ever been demonstrated in medicine, it is the fact, that tuberculosis, wherever we find it, is invariably produced by specific germs."[23]

As the society grew, it became increasingly impractical to have each member participate. With the appointment of a program committee in the mid-1890s, "the haphazard and irresponsible methods of the former years [gave] way to a scientific and well arranged plan of discussion."[24] Still, the program remained so crowded — over ninety papers were jammed into one session — that there was talk of either scheduling two parallel sections or limiting the number of papers. Most members favored the latter approach, and by the end of the century the annual session consisted of only thirty papers (twenty invited and ten volunteered), plus a few special addresses given by the president and distinguished nonmembers.[25] At last the society had a format conducive to scientific discourse.

In addition to discussing and publishing papers presented at the annual meetings, the society attempted to advance the cause of medical science by legal means. In the mid-1850s it created a committee to petition the legislature to legalize dissection for "the advancement of Anatomical and Surgical science." The governor in 1855 vetoed such a bill, and it was not until 1868 that the society finally obtained the protection it wanted. The new law not only legalized dissection, but stipulated:

It shall be the duty of each and every public officer having the charge of dead bodies, such as are required to be buried at the public expense, to deliver to any member or agent of a county or state medical society, each and every dead body of persons dying under his charge, unless within forty-eight hours after the death of such person or persons, the friends or relatives shall claim the same for interment.[26]

In 1871 the Winnebago County Medical Society asked the authorities in Oshkosh for the body of one John Hess, a deceased criminal, to be used for the "advancement of anatomical and surgical science."[27] Neither Hess's fate nor the law's contribution to medical science can be determined.

In an age notorious for its therapeutic controversies and quarrelsome physicians, the society's commitment "to cultivate harmony and kind feeling among the members of the Medical Profession" was laudable indeed.[28] For many members, the fellowship enjoyed at the annual sessions was the chief attraction of society membership. "We, at all times," recalled Dr. Sheldon, "emphasized the social element, and the Annual

Banquet and Smoker afforded an opportunity for making many new acquaintances and friends. We always had plenty of singing and the rousing chorus of 'The Saw-bones Choir' is still a joyous memory."[29] Minutes of the meetings are filled with praise for "tempting viands" and toasts that lasted late into the night. Sometimes the host physicians would add special excursions to the program, such as an afternoon of sailing on Lake Michigan or a concert in the park.[30]

The importance of these social events is illustrated by the nearly 50 percent drop in attendance one year after it was announced that there would be no banquet.[31] Some members, however, felt that the social program too often eclipsed the scientific, that the main attraction of the meetings should be "intellectual rather than gustatorial."[32] One physician in 1880 introduced a resolution banning future banquets on the grounds that "life is too short and too precious for us to run the risk of stuffing ourselves annually, as we have been in the habit heretofore of doing. . . . It takes up our time, it destroys our health, and in every way serves a bad purpose, rather than a good one." But his suggestion did not sit well with at least one of the less straitlaced members, who argued that "one of the great benefits of a State Medical Society is the cul-

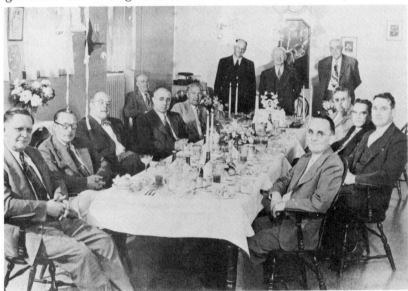

The Medical History of Langlade County, Wisconsin, 1880–1976
(Madison: Women's Auxiliary to the Langlade County Medical Society
and the State Medical Society of Wisconsin, 1976), p. 22

Social events, like this Langlade County Medical Society banquet, helped to maintain unity and good will among local physicians.

tivation of the social element, and the becoming better acquainted with each other, not only scientifically but socially."[33] Needless to say, the banquets continued.

For decades society fellowship seems to have been limited to white males, even though the association technically had no "tests of race, color, or sex." In fact, President John Favill in 1872 offered his "most cordial right hand" to "any woman of thorough medical education, and good character, who desires to devote herself to the practice of medicine." "St. Paul may have ruled her out of the pulpit," he said, "but St. Paul never did say that she would not make a 'good Samaritan.'"[34] Despite such sentiments, however, no woman joined the state society until 1885, sixteen years after Dr. Laura J. Ross broke the sex barrier of the Milwaukee Medical Society.[35]

Another way in which the society fostered professional harmony was by occasionally disciplining members whose actions had disturbed the profession's peace. This was done through the committee on ethics, established in 1872. During its first afternoon in existence the committee expelled a Milwaukee physician for converting to homeopathy and a Fond du Lac practitioner for public advertising.[36] But after this initial demonstration of intent, disciplinary action occurred infrequently and more often for offenses against the profession than against the public.[37]

In addition to its social and scientific functions, the State Medical Society of Wisconsin took a genuine interest in public health, broadly defined. At times its involvement may have stemmed from mixed motives, but there can be little doubt, I think, that the physicians of Wisconsin often had the public's interest at heart. President Edwin Bartlett expressed the prevailing sentiment in 1885:

A medical society affords the best opportunity to discuss and organize movements for the public good. . . . The employment of the color-blind, the best method of educating the deaf and dumb, the prevention of the pollution of the lakes and streams, and the prevention of preventable diseases, the construction of schoolhouses, the nature of inebriety and the most successful treatment for inebriates, insanity and the arrangement of insane asylums. All these are live questions of to-day that need immediate attention.[38]

On occasion the society even placed the public good above self-interest, at least in theory. In 1851 it adopted a resolution, introduced by Harmon Van Dusen, reminding members that when testifying in malpractice suits, "it is their duty respectively, as the conservators of the public health and the honor of the medical profession, to give unqualified, decided, and direct opinions, whether in favor of or against the medical or surgical practitioner who may be interested in the result of the suit."[39]

During its early years the society's public health activities were limited mainly to petitioning the state legislature for laws requiring "the Registration of Births, Marriages, Deaths, and principal diseases of each town in the State,"[40] prohibiting druggists from dispensing "poisons" without a physician's prescription,[41] and providing for "a State Lunatic Asylum" or, as the final resolution read, a "Hospital for the Insane." Behind this last motion, approved in 1856, was Dr. Alfred L. Castleman, a Milwaukee physician and entrepreneur, who clearly had conflicting interests. Although sympathetic to the needs of the mentally ill, he also hoped to get the state's business. Fortunately, the society rejected his proposal, and in 1860 a state-run Hospital for the Insane opened near Madison.[42]

The plight of the mentally ill remained a concern of the society throughout the nineteenth century. The occasional tours of the state mental institution, in conjunction with the annual meetings, always elicited considerable interest. At the request of the Association of Medical Superintendents of American Institutions for the Insane, the society in 1886 approved a resolution calling on Congress to control the number of "defective" immigrants, who were seen as "the chief cause" of the rapidly increasing incidence of insanity, pauperism, and crime in the country.[43] The following year the state's physicians took a more positive approach to the problems of mental illness by urging the legislature to appropriate $20,000 for the care of "idiots and feeble-minded," then often caged "like beasts" in local almshouses.[44] The society during the 1890s agitated for the passage of "just and humane laws" for the insane, especially a bill prohibiting the imprisonment of the insane pending commitment.[45]

The state medical society lost a chance to advance the cause of public health in the early 1870s when a special committee appointed to lobby for a state board of health "neglected to perform its duty." Thus credit for establishment of the state board in 1876 went instead to the Sauk County Medical Society, which secured passage of the necessary legislation.[46]

In the name of public health the state medical society repeatedly spoke out on two of the great moral questions of the day: abortion and obscenity. According to one member, abortion was an evil ten times greater than intemperance. "I do not believe," he told the society in 1870, "there is a single Physician present who doubts for a moment, that where one living child is born into the world, two are done away with by means of criminal abortion."[47] Already the society had taken an official stand on the issue, voting at the time of reorganization to expel any member guilty of performing criminal abortions, that is, abortions for nontherapeutic reasons. A year later the members vowed "to drive from

---

THE RESCUE HOME
BABCOCK, :-: WIS.

An ethical home and maternity hospital for unfortunate girls.

Situated in a quiet little village in the center of the state.

Private and Charity Cases received.

Secrecy is a fundamental principle of management.

The Medical Profession owes its support to this practical effort to circumvent the abortionist.

Following is one of a number of testimonials we have received.

Fox Lake, Wis., Feb. 5, 1908.

To whom it may concern:
I wish to say that it has been my experience to have to send an unfortunate girl to the institution known as "Our Rescue Home" at Babcock, Wis. That this girl's experience as well as treatment shown her mother in the sad ending of her case, has convinced me that the institution is deserving of the co-operation of the best Medical Men of this state and especially am I convinced the present manager, Mr. R. M. Clare, is a Man having the best interest of the institution at heart.   Sincerely,
                                       W. H. WATTERSON, M. D.

ADDRESS ALL CORRESPONDENCE TO
THE RESCUE HOME,
BABCOCK, :-: WIS.

Wisconsin Medical Journal 6 (1907–8): xxxi

As part of their campaign against illegal abortions, Wisconsin physicians supported homes for unwed mothers like this one in Babcock.

our midst any guilty member (if there be any such)," arguing that abortion was not only immoral but the cause of "a large number of diseases of the most dangerous character."[48]

The society, like medical bodies elsewhere, condemned obscenity — that is, sexually explicit language — with equal vigor. In the 1870s it created a committee on obscene medical literature to work for a law, similar to one in New York, banning the "circulation of obscene literature, illustrations, advertisements, and articles of indecent and immoral use, and obscene advertisements in Patent Medicines, &c." The committee, however, failed in its mission and disbanded after three years.[49] But the problem remained, and by the early 1900s this "villainy" was threatening the society "on all sides." The *Wisconsin Medical Journal* in 1904 directed the attention of "every honest and decency-loving individual" to

another evil . . . the filthy "manhood restored" columns of our daily press, illustrated in a manner to bring the blush of shame to every cheek, couched in terms that appeal to the lascivious element of developing youth, and detailing as afflictions certain conditions that are normal — and all this merely to exact tribute from those innocent enough to put credence in these foul and lying statements.[50]

Three years later the society announced that, partly as a result of its efforts, the legislature had just made it illegal for advertisers to refer to "any diseases pertaining to the sexual organs."[51]

In the opinion of Dr. C. S. Sheldon, one of the society's most important accomplishments "in the interest of public health" was its support in the late 1880s of a pre-medical course at the University of Wisconsin.[52] In one sense this is ironic, because throughout the nineteenth century the medical society strongly opposed the university's ambitions to train physicians, fearing perhaps, as many practitioners did, the competition of well-educated young doctors in an already overcrowded field. In 1850, two years after the legislature had authorized a medical department at the state university, Dr. Alfred Castleman, then president of the state medical society, met with the university chancellor to discuss a possible organization. Their conference, however, "resulted in reporting against the expediency of the immediate organization of said Department."[53] (The professorship of theory and practice of medicine, to which Castleman was appointed five years later, existed only on paper.) In 1868 the president of the university encouraged the medical society to take the initiative in organizing a medical school, but after two years of discussion the society concluded that such a venture was "not at present advisable."[54] It seemed even less advisable in 1875, when University President John Bascom proposed creating an intersectarian medical department, with equal privileges for homeopaths, eclectics, and allopaths. His suggestion to have "mixed Schools of Medicine" outraged the regulars, who once again insisted that a medical school was "inexpedient."[55] It was not until 1886 that the society, still somewhat suspicious of the university's intentions, agreed to support a course of preliminary medical studies — "it being understood that this is not to be a Medical Department in any sense of the word."[56]

Besides lobbying to improve the public health, the state medical society at times tried to educate the public and the profession regarding the importance of sanitation and preventive medicine. The theme of prevention frequently appears in the annual addresses of the presidents. "The highest duty of the physician is not to cure disease, but to prevent it," declared J. B. Whiting in 1876.[57] "The mission of the physician today," echoed J. K. Bartlett the next year, is "to teach how illness may be avoided and prevented. . . . The individual and the community must be taught that all epidemic, endemic, and contagious diseases which scourge humanity, are but direct results of violation of health laws; and that they are either preventable in their nature, or can be cut short in their devastations by means, now to a great extent, understood."[58]

The society's efforts at health education became more formalized shortly after the turn of the century, when state and county committees on public health and hygiene were established to provide the public with practical information on sanitation, preventive medicine, and personal hygiene. In this way the society hoped to "become a center of instruction and beneficience to the whole community" while at the same time "restoring prestige with the public at large," thus felicitously combining public service with professional advancement.[59]

The same mixture of altruism and self-interest can be seen in the society's efforts "to protect ourselves and society against the imposition of medical pretenders," although in this instance the physicians probably had substantially more to gain (in terms of reduced competition) than their patients. Given the poor quality of regular medicine in the nineteenth century and the relatively harmless treatments of many sectarians, the people of Wisconsin scarcely suffered more at the hands of irregulars than regulars. Of course, they also had to contend with outright mountebanks and quacks.

The state medical society's first recorded attempt to deal with the problem of irregular practitioners dates from 1850, when it appointed physicians in each county to take a census of the various types of individuals practicing medicine. The plan failed, however, when "in many cases irregulars were appointed, and as a consequence irregulars would be reported as graduates, quacks as doctors, and so on."[60] In 1869, in response to a recommendation by the American Medical Association, the society voted to create a board of censors to examine physicians entering the state, but this was a purely extralegal measure.[61] It was not until the late 1870s, with the appointment of a special committee "to consider the best means for preventing quackery and to prevent unqualified persons from practicing medicine in the state," that the society began making "very strenuous" legal efforts to restrict the practice of medicine to regularly trained physicians like themselves.[62]

In justifying the need for licensing laws, self-conscious society members repeatedly assured one another than their sole concern was the protection of the public, daily robbed "in pocket and life" by the "unqualified" physicians of the state, estimated to be at least 50 percent of all practitioners.[63] "We stand between the people and disease and suffering," said one member. "It is the people we want to protect, and not ourselves."[64] Perhaps so, but at least a few members felt otherwise. "I am pleased to note that the founders of our Society were frank enough to admit that they, not the public alone, wanted some protection," said the president of the society in 1899. "Let it be understood, that while all measures directed against medical pretenders cannot but result primarily and chiefly in the good and protection of the general public, yet, if any aid or protection can be given the medical profession, it is fully entitled to the same, and let us not be too modest to ask for it."[65]

So great was its desire for a licensing law that the State Medical Soci-

ety of Wisconsin deigned to collaborate even with its traditional arch-
enemies, the Homeopathic Medical Society of the State of Wisconsin
and the Wisconsin State Eclectic Medical Society, which represented
the two largest and best educated medical sects. The homeopathic society, organized in 1865 and incorporated three years later, listed 76
members in 1880, compared with 181 active members in the regular
society.[66] The eclectic society, the smallest of the three, had been in existence since 1870.[67] For decades the regulars had branded the homeopaths and eclectics as "medical pretenders," and their code of ethics still
prohibited professional consultations with these sectarians.

In the fall of 1879 Nicholas Senn and other members of the committee
on medical legislation met in Milwaukee with homeopathic and eclectic
representatives to draft a bill creating a state board of medical examiners. Surprisingly, the three parties soon reached agreement on a measure
calling for a seven-man board composed of four regulars, two homeopaths, and one eclectic.[68] Their proposal died in the legislature, although the lawmakers did approve a bill in 1881 restricting use of "the
title of doctor, physician, or surgeon, by means of any abbreviation, or
by the use of any word or words," to persons holding medical school diplomas or membership in a state or county medical society. This was
admittedly a small gain, but, suggested Secretary Reeve hopefully, perhaps it would serve as "an entering wedge . . . to a better law in the
future."[69]

As more and more midwestern states passed licensing laws, Wisconsin increasingly became a dumping ground for physicians unqualified
to practice elsewhere — "the chosen field of quacks and charlatans without number."[70] Thus the state medical society in the late 1880s and early
1890s stepped up its efforts to obtain protective legislation.[71] It was not,
however, until 1897 — fully a decade after neighboring states like Iowa,
Illinois, and Minnesota had enacted similar laws — that the state legislators passed the long-sought-for measure. The Wisconsin law called for
the creation of a state board of medical examiners, composed of three
regulars, two homeopaths, and two eclectics, recommended by the respective medical societies and appointed by the governor. To prevent a
medical monopoly, five affirmative votes were necessary to approve a
license.[72] The legislature amended this law in 1901 to provide for osteopathic representation on the board and to require a diploma from a
four-year medical school.[73]

Wisconsin's delay in passing a medical licensing law is not easily explained. Among both regulars and sectarians, some physicians feared
requirements so high that they might prevent tolerably competent individuals from practicing medicine.[74] Others simply felt that the public

did not need protection. The people "can protect themselves," argued Dr. William Fox of Milwaukee, "by choosing a doctor in good standing, and who is not a quack."[75] A few blamed the state's leading newspapers, particularly the *Milwaukee Sentinel*, for the delay. According to the chairman of the committee on medical legislation, the *Sentinel* prostituted itself soley for "the revenue which it derives from quack doctors, mountebanks, and patent medicine men."[76] But this economic interpretation failed to convince at least one prominent member of the state society, who pointed out that the newspaper was probably motivated by a genuine concern that the law might give "unequal advantage to some one or more of the several schools of practice."[77]

The fact that Wisconsin dentists won licensing legislation twelve years before physicians achieved that objective suggests that the legislature did not oppose licensing in principle. Organized in 1870, the Wisconsin State Dental Society pledged itself to protect "the public from the evils of empiricism," otherwise known as quackery. The entire dental profession had been brought into disrepute, declared one speaker at the society's 1875 meeting, by "abominable quacks who disgrace the name of 'dentist' to say nothing of the term 'doctor' they so delight to affix to their names." One self-proclaimed practitioner bragged that "any man who could make a hoe-handle could make a set of teeth," while another reportedly abandoned mule driving to take up the practice of dentistry. Although some reputable dentists opposed restrictive legislation to prevent such abuses, others saw licensing as the only solution. Like many physicians, the latter insisted that they sought to protect the public, not to gain competitive advantage. "Do we suffer?" asked one. "No, it is the people, and they should be protected." After a comparatively short debate the legislature approved the creation of a state board of dental examiners in 1885.[78] The reasons for the dentists' early victory remain unclear, but the absence of sectarian divisions within dentistry, the proven efficacy of dental practice, and the political sophistication of the dentists may all have been contributing factors.[79]

During the nineteenth century, and especially in the last few decades, scores of independent local medical societies sprang up throughout the state. A handful grew so large and influential that they retarded the development of the state medical society,[80] but most died in infancy, leaving scarcely a trace for the twentieth-century historian.[81] We do know, however, of various county, regional, ethnic, and sectarian societies, as well as groups devoted primarily to the advancement of science, like the Milwaukee Academy of Medicine, founded in 1886. One or two medical societies were purely social, if not hedonistic. The A. C. Club in Milwaukee, for example, seems to have done little besides sponsor revelrous annual picnics, described as "genial gathering[s] for the sole purpose of jollification, even carousal."[82]

Of greater significance were the local medical societies operating under territorial or state charter. Milwaukee boasted a medical society as early as 1837, but its first legally incorporated one was apparently the Milwaukee Medical Society, created in 1846 by 28 county physicians.[83] The regular practitioners of Dane County organized a similar society four years later. Both groups struggled for years to stay alive, and in 1857 the Madison physicians changed their name to the Wisconsin Central Medical Association and annexed eleven neighboring counties. But even this act of imperialism failed to bring out more than five or six members to the association's meetings.[84] An incomplete American Medical Association survey in 1873 found only six regular medical societies besides the Wisconsin State Medical Society: the Rock River Medical Society, with 11 active members, the Waupaca County Medical Society (12), the Winnebago County Medical Society (35), the Fond du Lac Medical Society (32), the Milwaukee Medical Society (11), and the Racine Medical Association, whose membership was unknown.[85] By 1902 regular physicians in Wisconsin were operating ten county and five regional medical societies recognized by the state association.[86]

Local societies, even more than the state body, tended to be inward looking, focusing principally on professional rather than social issues. An examination of the minutes of various local societies reveals that members channeled most of their limited energies into three areas: economics, ethics, and medical science. For most societies, one of the first acts after writing a constitution was drawing up a fee bill setting minimum rates for services, "it being understood that the fee may properly be increased in any given case, and especially where the responsibility is great."[87] These fee schedules were often printed and prominently displayed during the nineteenth century, but later they became less visible and sometimes secret. Although most county society constitutions banned fee bills after 1903, this prohibition seems to have been honored primarily in the breach.[88]

Some societies kept a "dead beat list" or "black list" of patients delinquent in paying their bills. The Winnebago County Medical Society in 1869 requested each member "to contribute toward a Black List by giving to the Secretary the names and residence of those persons, who can but through dishonesty will not remunerate physicians for professional services rendered." The purpose of the list was "to exclude all such persons from medical attendance until such time as the said person or persons shall give satisfactory evidence of honesty as will enable the proposer to strike such name from the list."[89] The businesslike physicians of

PHYSICIANS' FEE BILL.

At a meeting of the Physicians of Waukesha County, held at the house of A. L. Castleman, on the 16th day of December, 1846, Doctor Jno. R. Goodno' was called to the chair, and A. L. Castleman was appointed Secretary.

On motion of Dr. Warren, the following was adopted, as the fee-bill of the physicians subscribing thereto:

Ordinary Office Prescription,..............$0,50
Bloodletting, Extracting Teeth, &c..............25
Opening Abscess, ad. lib.,.....................50
Vaccination, (not exceeding 3 in a family,) each,..50
Cupping,.....................................1,00
Introducing Seaton or Issue,................1,00
Verbal Advice,.............................0,50
Letter of Advice,....................$1 to 5,00
Ordinary Visits,.........................1,00
Night Visits,..............................1,50
Additional patients, same fam., not exceeding one,.50
  "   "   "   " all above one, each.25
Consultation,..............................3,00
Obstetrical Attendance,.....☞CASH☜1....5,00
  "   "   " called after Midwife,$10 to 30,00
Twin Cases,................"......"........8,00
Instrumental Labour,......."......"......10,00
Semi-obstetrical Attendance,.."......"......3,00
Mileage, ...(in night, 75 cts., per mile,)......50
Gonorrhoea,...(to be paid in advance,).......5,00
Syphilis,........."......."...............10,00
Introducing Catheter,....(first time,)..·····..3,00
Succeeding Introductions,..................1,00
Operation for Hydrocele,...................5,00
Excision of Tonsils,.....................10,00
Paracentesis Abdominis,...................5,00

Operations for Phimosis or Paraphimosis....5,00
  "..........".....Fistula Lachrymalis,25,00
  "..........".....Hare Lip,.........10,00
  "..........".....Hernia,...........50,00
Reducing Hernia,..........................5,00
  "....Prolapsus Uteri,.................3,00
Operation for imperfarate Anus or Vagina,....10,00
  "....". Fistula in Ano,..............25,00
Dividing Fraenum Linguae, or Penis,.........1,00
Tying Arteries for Aneurism, ad. lib.........25,00
Trephining,...............................50,00
Dressing Cataract,.........................50,00
Operation for Strabismus,..................10,00
Extirpating Eye,.........................100,00
Operation for Club Foot,..................25,00
Reducing Simple Fracture of Thigh,.......15,00
  "......"......"....Leg or Arm,.....10,00
  "......"......Dislocation of Thigh,...15,00
  "......"......"..Shoulder or Wrist,..5,00
  "......"......"..Ankle,...........10,00
Amputating Thigh, Leg or Foot,...........50,00
  ".....Finger or Toe,.................5,00
  ".....Arm, Fore-arm or Wrist,.......25,00
  ".....Hip or Shoulder Joint,..$50 to 100,00
Extirpate Breast,.........................35,00
  "....Testicle, ...25,00

RESOLVED—That we will *honorably,* and in *good faith* maintain the rates of our fee-bill, and adhere in practice to its *specific items,* as a compensation for our services; Provided, however, that we will make a deduction of 20 per cent on all sums paid within 60 days after service is rendered, except for obstetrical attendance.

RESOLVED—That we will settle our account for professional services, by note or otherwise, *annually,* by the first day of January.

JNO. R. GOODNO',
A. L. CASTLEMAN,
H. B. TOWNSEND,
Wm. H. WARNER,

D. H. SHUMWAY,
P. M. HACKLEY Jr.,
A. J. STOREY,
J. JOHNSTONE.,

In 1846 a group of physicians in Waukesha County agreed to charge uniform rates for their services and drew up one of the earliest surviving fee bills in Wisconsin.

Oshkosh also resolved that year to hire a bill collector—preferably a local preacher—to recover overdue accounts.[90]

Besides regulating and collecting fees, some county societies tried to equalize competition by controlling members' office hours. The Brown County Medical Society, for example, at one time required members to confine their evening practices to Mondays, Wednesdays, and Saturdays, and in 1920 seriously discussed "the advisability of adjusting afternoon office hours for the convenience of golfers."[91]

The local groups of physicians devoted much time—perhaps too much time—to disciplining members who violated medical etiquette by advertising, stealing patients, gossiping about a "brother physician," entering the saloon business, or merely consulting with a sectarian. After reviewing two decades of debates in the Milwaukee City Medical Association, Dr. Louis F. Frank lamented "the all too numerous petty quarrels and accusations of individual members for alleged interference in practice, consultations with expelled members and adherents of other doctrines."[92]

Local physicians spent considerable time presenting and discussing clinical cases, but their reports were often perfunctory and of little scientific value. From time to time county societies did advise their communities on public health matters like sanitation, the purity of water and milk, and measures to take against epidemics, but their counsel, though well intentioned, may occasionally have done more harm than good. During the 1849 cholera epidemic the Milwaukee City Medical Association resolved

that no fact in medicine, in the opinion of this association, is more clearly determined than that the Asiatic Cholera is not contagious, and any action on the part of the authorities which is based upon the supposition that it is so, and subjects the sick to any inconvenience, is clearly unwarrantable and inhuman, and will not receive the sanction of any of its members.[93]

The Wisconsin Central Medical Association attempted in 1865 to settle the contagionist-anticontagionist controversy, because "all agreed that it was politic for medical men to talk alike" on such matters. Unfortunately, the outcome is not known.[94]

Despite their many imperfections, nineteenth-century local medical societies undoubtedly improved the morale and public image of physicians. One example will suffice. When Dr. Alexander Schue arrived in Madison in 1855, he found the profession rent with discord and jealousy. Scarcely a year later, after resuscitating the Dane County Medical Society, he was able to tell a friend: "There is in general much good feeling manifest between the members of the profession here, fostered as it undoubtably is through the agency of a medical society which was organized and called into existence by my efforts."[95] If it accomplished no more, the society had proved its worth.

Wisconsin's local medical societies operated independently of the state society—and occasionally at cross-purposes. This, of course, reduced the effectiveness of both organizations. It was not until 1903 that state and county societies joined to form one organic whole. The merger grew out of a nationwide movement, begun in 1901 with the reorganization of the American Medical Association. At its annual session that year the AMA approved a plan requiring all of its members to join their respective county and state societies. It also created a House of Delegates, made up of representatives from constituent state societies, and encouraged the state associations to set up similar legislative bodies, composed of county society delegates. In 1902 the committee on reorganization of the State Medical Society of Wisconsin endorsed the AMA's proposal for a unified county-state-national federation, arguing that a strong alliance was necessary "in order that we may have proper protection and wield our just share of power in scientific and political affairs in the State and Nation."[96]

But some Wisconsin physicians thought otherwise. The president of the state medical society himself declared it "most unjust" to require members of that body to join the frequently inferior county organizations. In his opinion, such coercion would only reduce the size of the state medical society, which already claimed less than one-third of eligible physicians.[97] Equally suspicious of the plan were the large regional societies, like those in central Wisconsin and the Fox River Valley, which feared extinction as newly organized county societies drew off their members.[98] To further complicate the situation, two societies in Milwaukee County began feuding over which one was legally entitled to represent that area's physicians.[99]

Dr. J. N. McCormack of Kentucky, the AMA's official organizer, arrived in Wisconsin in March 1903 to bring the state's recalcitrant physicians into line. His visit was a complete success.[100] At its annual session in June the State Medical Society of Wisconsin became the twenty-third state society in the nation to embrace reorganization.[101] By late summer twenty existing or newly created county societies were requesting recognition by the state body, and "Medical Society Spirit"—to use Secretary Sheldon's favorite phrase—was fast gaining ground.[102] Within a year membership more than doubled, from 630 to 1,311, and by 1915 Wisconsin boasted the highest membership percentage (73 percent) of any state in the union, far surpassing its sister societies in Iowa, Illinois, and Minnesota.[103]

To complete the unification of the medical profession, regular societies in 1903 opened their doors to reputable sectarian practitioners,
whom fifty years earlier they had ostracized as "medical pretenders."
But times — and practices — had changed. Since the late 1870s the regulars had been working harmoniously with homeopaths and eclectics on
licensing legislation, and by the close of the century the once-sharp
therapeutic differences among the schools were beginning to fade. In
his 1894 presidential address, B. C. Brett urged conciliation. "While we
should prefer to mingle with those of our own faith," he said, "we
should not harbor feelings of contempt for educated gentlemen of other
schools."[104] A few years later C. S. Sheldon observed that the old antag-
onisms seemed to be disappearing:

The regular profession is disposed to adopt a broader and more liberal policy toward our sectarian brethren. . . . this is a wise departure and in no sense a lowering of our standards. Come what may, we may all agree that character, education, and ability should be the final tests of eligibility. Moreover, it would be
well if we might be more concerned in excluding the unworthy and incompetent
in our own ranks, than in putting up barriers against the admission of good men
outside the regular profession.[105]

On the eve of reorganization approximately 2500 licensed physicians
were practicing in Wisconsin: 80.6 percent regulars, 14.0 percent homeopaths, 3.4 percent eclectics, and 2.0 percent osteopaths.[106] Under
the new constitution adopted by county societies, all of these practitioners became eligible for membership — provided that they were "of good
moral and professional standing" and did not "claim to practice sectarian medicine."[107] For a year or two the regular societies required incoming homeopaths and eclectics (there is no mention of osteopaths) to
sever all ties with their traditional organizations, but in 1905 they cast
off this last shackle of "an unnatural prejudice" and began actively re-
cruiting their former rivals.[108] This proved to be the kiss of death for the
sectarian societies. "Our State Society is not as well attended as it should
be," lamented Wisconsin homeopaths in 1906, "due to the fact that so
many of our homeopathic physicians are affiliating with the County,
State and National Societies of the old school, something which is very
much to be deplored."[109]

The reorganized State Medical Society of Wisconsin, backed by its
county constituents, turned out to be particularly effective in representing the political and economic interests of the profession. Though it
continued to cultivate a fraternal spirit, to contribute to the public
health, and to promote the advancement and dissemination of medical
science, nonclinical issues — from malpractice to "socialized medicine"

Physicians Business Association of Sheboygan

MINIMUM FEE SCHEDULE
ADOPTED JANUARY 12TH, 1920

General Practice

Day visits in city or at Hospital	$ 3.00
Emergency calls or calls made during office hours	5.00
Night visits received and made after 9 P. M. and before 7 A. M.	5.00
Ordinary day consultation in City	5.00
Subsequent joint attendance in City	3.00
Consultation in City (not confinements) at night 9 P. M. to 7 A. M.	10.00
Country Consultation. (Day)	5.00 and mileage
Country consultation. (Night)	10.00 and mileage
Office or telephone consultation.	1.00
Country visits. (Day) $1.00 per mile plus	3.00
Country visits. (Night) $1.00 per mile plus	10.00
Physical examination of the chest or abdomen	2.00
Written opinion on a case. (not medico-legal)	5.00
Certificate of health	2.00
Vaccination at office	1.00
Vaccination at home	3.00
Each additional vaccination at home	1.00
Fitting Truss	2.00
Life Insurance Examination	5.00
Visits at Kohler, Wis. (Day)	5.00
Visits at Kohler, Wis. (Night)	7.50
Accompanying patient out of the city. (per day or fraction thereof)	50.00 and expenses
Administering anesthetic. Major operation	10.00
Minor operation	5.00
Visiting patient for the purpose of giving testimony in court	10.00
Post mortem examination. Viewing body	5.00
Filling out accident or sick benefit blanks	1.00
Examination of urine. (Chemical)	3.00
" " (Microscopical)	3.00
" " sputum	2.00
" " blood	3.00
Administering prophylactic serums and vaccines	2.00
Administering Arsphenamine or Neo-Arsphenamine	20.00
Intra-muscular administration of Mercury	3.00
X-Ray treatments	3.00
Radiographs. (Trunk or extremities)	5.00
" (Dental)	3.00
Spinal puncture	25.00
Introducing catheters, sounds or bougies	2.00
Post-mortems requiring autopsy	25.00
Rectal examination for diagnosis or treatment	2.00

SURGERY

Fractures

Reduction and first dressing: Fracture of the Femur	$ 75.00
Subsequent dressing of the Femur	2.00
Reduction and first dressing Fracture of leg below knee	50.00
" " " " " arm below elbow	50.00
" " " " " arm above elbow	50.00
" " " " " arm involving elbow joint	50.00
" " " " " small bones	10.00
" " " " " jaw	25.00
" " " " " clavicle	25.00
" " " " " rib	10.00

Compound or comminuted fractures, 25% additional will be charged.

Dislocations

Reducing dislocation of hip	$ 75.00
" " " shoulder	25.00
" " " elbow or knee	25.00
" " " ankle or wrist	25.00
" " " jaw	10.00
" " " of other joints	5.00

Amputations

Amputation of arm or forearm	$ 75.00
" " leg or thigh	75.00
" " thigh at hip joint	100.00
" " arm at shoulder joint	100.00
" " fingers or toes	10.00

Resections

Resections of large bones or joints	100.00
" " small	25.00
Application of casts	10.00

Operations

Major operations such as, Appendectomy, Cholecystotomy, Herniotomy, Hysterectomy, Salpingectomy, Nephrotomy or Nephrectomy, Prostatectomy, Cystotomy, Removal of Breast or Abdominal tumors, Trephining Skull and Skull Fractures, Uterine suspension and all other operations of similar degree of severity and magnitude.	$100.00
Enucleation of eye, Iridectomy, Mastoidectomy, Tracheotomy and operation for Cataract	100.00
Operation for Varicocele and Hydrocele	75.00
" " Talipes	50.00
" " Hemorroids, Fistula in Ano, and Anal Fissure	50.00
" " Hare lip or Cleft Palate	50.00
" " Extirpation of Testicle	50.00
" " Extirpation of Tonsils	25.00
Resection of rib for Empyema	50.00
Removal of polypus, Nasal or Rectal	25.00
Tenotomy	25.00
Phymosis or Paraphymosis	25.00
Paracentesis: Thorax, Abdomen, Bladder or Hydrocele	10.00
Reducing Hernia by Taxis	10.00
Removal of ingrown toe nails	15.00
Ligating arteries (Small)	10.00
" " (Large)	25.00
Minor operations, suturing of small wounds, etc.	$ 5.00
Removal of foreign bodies from eye, ear or nose	2.00
Assisting in Major operation	10.00
Assisting in Minor operation	5.00

Obstetrics and Gynecology

Ordinary obstetrical delivery and four extra visits	$ 25.00
Instrumental delivery or version	35.00
Delivery of placenta	10.00
Vaginal examination for diagnosis or treatment	2.00
Curetting uterus	35.00
Operation for lacerated perineun	100.00
Operation for lacerated cervix	50.00
Operation for Vesico-Vaginal or Vesico-Rectal Fistula	100.00
Removal of Uterine polyp	25.00
Reduction of inverted uterus	50.00

These charges are for the performance of the operation only. Assistants fees and subsequent visits are additional. The fee for surgical dressings depend on the quantity and quality of the dressings required.

For operations and services not enumerated above, charges will be made according to their nature, extent, importance, skill required and the responsibility involved.

DIX PRINTING COMPANY

Department of the History of Medicine, University of Wisconsin–Madison

Fee schedules reflected changing economic conditions as well as therapeutic practices. These rates are part of a minimum fee schedule adopted by the Physicians Business Association of Sheboygan in 1920.

—increasingly absorbed its attention.[110] At the same time an array of newly formed specialty societies, devoted almost exclusively to clinical medicine, partially freed the state medical society from its earlier scientific responsibilities, allowing it to concentrate more on solving the problems created by rising medical costs and increasing demands for health care services.[111] In responding to these problems, the society once again wrestled with the perennial question of its primary allegiance: to the public or to the profession.

The passage of the workmen's compensation law in 1911 convinced many Wisconsin physicians that they could no longer remain aloof from the pressing social reforms of the day. Since the medical profession had scarcely participated in the discussions leading up to the passage of workmen's compensation, it was "merely a matter of good fortune" that the legislation was not inimical to the interests of the profession. In the future, however, the physicians determined to "lead and not be led."[112]

A welcome opportunity to do so came in 1915, when the issue of compulsory health insurance first appeared on the horizon. At the annual meeting of the state medical society that year President T. J. Redelings urged his colleagues to spearhead the movement toward state medicine, arguing that since only 5 percent of American families could readily afford adequate medical care, compulsory health insurance was essential.[113] Surprisingly, many Wisconsin physicians agreed with this opinion, and the next year the House of Delegates voted *unanimously* to "commend the principle of compulsory health insurance and [to] pledge our support in the inactment of this principle into law."[114] In taking this bold step, the State Medical Society of Wisconsin became one of only two state medical societies in the nation to endorse compulsory health insurance.[115] This phase of the insurance movement collapsed shortly thereafter, but for a brief period the doctors of Wisconsin stood unequivocally for the public interest.

During the Great Depression in the 1930s, when economic disaster struck physicians and patients alike, the issue of health insurance reappeared. This time two possibilities were being discussed: voluntary as well as compulsory. The state medical society greeted the former with suspicion, the latter with downright hostility. In 1935 it officially disapproved of any nonsociety plans for providing voluntary insurance to low-income groups. In defiance of this decision, several Milwaukee physicians the very next year independently organized the Milwaukee Health Center, which offered unlimited medical and surgical services to the employees of the International Harvester Company for a monthly fee of $1.00 per man or $3.00 per family. On March 30, 1936, the Milwaukee County Medical Society expelled the participating physicians on charges of violating the code of ethics, which banned the solicitation of patients and contract practice. Both the state medical society and the American Medical Association upheld the expulsion — to their great embarrassment a few years later, when the affair received national publicity during the AMA's trial (resulting in conviction) for violating the Sherman Anti-Trust Act.[116]

But Wisconsin's physicians were not as hostile to voluntary health insurance as this one episode might suggest. Nor were they unconcerned about the welfare of the public. When Assemblyman Andrew J. Biemiller of Milwaukee in 1937 introduced bills calling for statewide compulsory health insurance and health cooperatives, the president of the state medical society issued a statement saying:

The one and only yardstick that will be used by the medical profession in evaluating these bills and determining its attitude is the effect that this legislative action would have upon the public health. . . . The question of economic welfare and security for the medical profession, of course, cannot at any time enter into the picture. . . . We naturally do not care to be impoverished, and would not cheerfully welcome such a development. Neither do we seek increased affluence if it means a poorer quality of medical care. But I am quite sure we would willingly sacrifice any material advantages and support the entire program of socialized medicine if we feel that such a program would benefit the health of the people of the state of Wisconsin. . . . our one real and great concern in the whole problem is entirely in the interest of the prevention and cure of disease. All other things are secondary.[117]

To deal with these issues, the state medical society created a special committee to study the distribution of health services in Wisconsin. A year and several studies later, the committee recommended that the society itself sponsor health-insurance trials in three counties: Douglas, Milwaukee, and Rock. These experiments continued until the United States entered the war in 1941.[118]

With the coming of peace the state medical society entered the health-insurance business on a grand scale, creating the Wisconsin Plan in 1945 and the Wisconsin Physicians Service a year later. Under the Wisconsin Plan, "the nation's first medical society sponsored voluntary plan operated through private insurance carriers,"[119] the society merely approved minimum standards for commercially sold medical and surgical insurance. But the Wisconsin Physicians Service, a Blue Shield plan, was considerably more ambitious. Owned and operated by the state medical society itself, this "prodigious child" was soon providing surgical, maternity, and medical coverage for hundreds of thousands of Wisconsin residents.[120] As a result of these ventures, the secretary of the society could justifiably claim in 1954 that no other state medical society in America had "taken a more active part in the affairs of prepaid plans."[121]

The society's enthusiastic adoption of voluntary health insurance in the 1940s resulted from several influences. Of great importance was the specter of "socialized medicine," which terrified many physicians. To such individuals, it seemed "better to inaugurate a voluntary payment plan rather than wait for a state controlled plan."[122] But just as important as the threat of compulsory health insurance was the promise of better incomes and improved health care.[123] Health insurance, on the one hand, "would do away with the uncollectible accounts of doctors and hospitals. It would offer to the physician an opportunity of earning a living commensurate with the value of the service that he performs."[124] On the other hand, it allowed physicians to provide high-quality medical care for low-income families. The state medical society's health-insurance plans thus benefited both the public and the profession. As the society reported after a decade in the business, they "have been a stabilizing influence on physicians' incomes. They are a boon to the public because they provide a device for economical financing of major health care costs while preserving the patient's free choice of physician."[125] Again, public protection and self-interest had blended nicely.

By the mid-1970s the state medical society's concern with social and economic issues was greater than ever, as evidenced in part by the size of its staff working in these areas. Since 1923, when the society opened its first office and employed George Crownhart as its first full-time secretary,[126] the staff had grown to hundreds, the majority of whom handled the society's insurance interests. In 1975, as part of its first major organizational change in four decades, the society created the Physicians Alliance "to protect, promote and achieve the socioeconomic interests of the members of the State Medical Society of Wisconsin"—"with militancy if necessary."[127] Of course the state's physicians had no intention of accomplishing this at the public's expense. As the society's late secretary, Charles Crownhart, George Crownhart's brother and successor, put it: "There is nothing for the benefit of medicine unless it is for the benefit of the people. The two interests are identical."[128]

Notes

I wish to thank Jennifer Latham, Deanna Reed Springall, and Susan Schultz for their assistance in the preparation of this chapter.

1 *Madge E. Pickard and R. Carlyle Buley, The Midwest Pioneer: His Ills, Cures, & Doctors* (New York: Henry Schuman, 1946), pp. 159–60. By 1868, however, one Wisconsin physician was complaining that it was virtually

impossible to say anything new, because "our country is weekly, semi-monthly, monthly and quarterly, supplied with medical publications that give to the profession any new discoveries or improvements almost as soon as made"; *Transactions of the Wisconsin State Medical Society* 2 (1868): 42–43. Hereafter the title *Transactions* stands for both *Transactions of the Wisconsin State Medical Society* (1867–1879) and *Transactions of the State Medical Society of Wisconsin* (1880–1902).

2 F. Garvin Davenport and Katye Lou Davenport, "Practicing Medicine in Madison, 1855–57: Alexander Schue's Letters to Robert Peter," *Wisconsin Magazine of History* 26 (1942): 83–84.

3 On American medical societies, see W. B. McDaniel II, "A Brief Sketch of the Rise of American Medical Societies," in *History of American Medicine*, ed. Felix Marti-Ibañez (New York: MD Publications, 1959), pp. 133–41.

4 *Laws of the Territory of Wisconsin Passed at Madison by the Legislative Assembly* (Madison: W. W. Wyman, 1841), pp. 121–26. The society apparently granted only one diploma, to Coryden S. Farr of Prairie du Sac in 1858. *Transactions* 15 (1881): 50.

5 *Laws of the Territory of Wisconsin*, pp. 124–26; *Proceedings of the Wisconsin State Medical Society* (1855), p. 12 (hereafter cited as *Proceedings*).

6 Although there are no records extant for the period prior to 1847, there are indications that the first county society delegates attended in 1849; *Proceedings* (1855), pp. 8, 12.

7 John Favill, "On the Relations the Profession Holds and Ought to Hold towards Community," *Transactions* 6 (1872): 28.

8 Henry Baird Favill, "Early Medical Days in Wisconsin," in *Henry Baird Favill, 1860–1916*, ed. John Favill (Chicago: privately printed, 1917), p. 604; *Transactions* 20 (1886): 241.

9 *Proceedings* (1855), pp. 6, 11–12. There is no evidence to support McDaniel's claim that the organization of the American Medical Association in 1847 revitalized the Wisconsin State Medical Society; McDaniel, "Brief Sketch," p. 140.

10 *Proceedings* (1855), pp. 12–13; *Proceedings* (1856), p. 38. See also W. H. Brisbane to H. R. Storer, March 19, 1859, quoted in James C. Mohr, *Abortion in America: The Origins and Evolution of National Policy, 1800–1900* (New York: Oxford University Press, 1978), p. 151.

11 *Transactions* 2 (1868): 5, 23.

12 Ibid., pp. 24–25; *Transactions* 20 (1886): 241.

13 *Transactions* 5 (1871): 193–97.

14 *Transactions* 29 (1895): 26; C. S. Sheldon, "Annual Address of the President," *Wisconsin Medical Journal* 13 (1914–15): 176.

15 *Proceedings* (1855), p. 9 (appendix).

16 *Proceedings* (1856), p. 41; *Transactions* 4 (1870): 41.

17 *Proceedings* (1855), p. 18; *Proceedings* (1856), p. 9; *Transactions* 2 (1868): 62; *Transactions* 11 (1877): 13.

18 *Transactions* 2 (1868): 87–88. The society in the following years added other specialized committees.

19 J. A. Bach, "Some Things I Remember," *Milwaukee Medical Times*, December 1934, p. 20; *Transactions* 15 (1881): 45.

20 Howard A. Kelly, *A Cyclopedia of American Medical Biography*, 2 vols. (Philadelphia: W. B. Saunders Co., 1912), 2: 357–58.

21 See, e.g., N. Senn, "Recent Progress in Surgery," *Transactions* 15 (1881): 76; and "The Pathology and Morbid Anatomy of Tubercle," *Transactions* 16 (1882): 43.

22 *Transactions* 15 (1881): 24–25.

23 *Transactions* 18 (1884): 25.

24 *Transactions* 29 (1895): 25.

25 *Transactions* 32 (1898): x–xiii, 21–24; 33 (1899): ix, 23, 41.

26 *Proceedings* (1855), pp. 17, 23; *Transactions* 2 (1868): 51; *Transactions* 4 (1870): 66–67; William Snow Miller, "Early Efforts of the Wisconsin State Medical Society to Legalize Dissection," *Wisconsin Medical Journal* 34 (1935): 853–58.

27 Minutes, Winnebago County Medical Society, March 2, 1871, Wisconsin State Historical Society, Madison, Wis.

28 *Proceedings* (1855): 9 (appendix).

29 Fred L. Holmes, "Medical Practice Sixty Years Ago and Today: Dr. C. S. Sheldon, Madison, Secretary of State Medical Society for a Quarter of a Century, Reminisces on Life, Doctors and Patients," *Wisconsin Medical Journal* 25 (1926): 20.

30 *Transactions* 4 (1870): 40; 15 (1881): 47.

31 *Transactions* 14 (1880): 69.

32 *Transactions* 10 (1876): 29.

33 *Transactions* 14 (1880): 66–69.

34 John Favill, "On the Relations," p. 28.

35 *Transactions* 19 (1885): 71; Dennis H. Phillips, "Women in Nineteenth Century Wisconsin Medicine," *Wisconsin Medical Journal* 71 (1972): 13.

36 *Transactions* 6 (1872): 13, 15–16.

37 See, e.g., *Transactions* 17 (1883): 22–23.

38 Edwin Bartlett, "Fraternally Yours," *Transactions* 19 (1885): 154.

39 *Transactions* 2 (1868): 13.

40 Ibid., pp. 11–13, 16. In 1856 the secretary of the society reprimanded some members for complaining that the registration law eventually passed "imposes upon them much labor without recompense," and he reminded them that they were the "conservators of the public health"; *Proceedings* (1856), p. 39.

41 *Transactions* 3 (1869): 5–6. One member argued that "there was a general incompetency among druggists. . . . Accidents are frequent and the public need protection"; ibid., p. 5. For a later, less negative view of pharmacists, see *Transactions* 29 (1895): 11–12.

42 *Proceedings* (1856), pp. 6, 43–47 (appendix); Donald R. McNeil, "Dr. Alfred L. Castleman, Agitator and Critic," *Wisconsin Medical Journal* 51 (1952): 293.

43 *Transactions* 20 (1886): 34–35.

44 *Transactions* 21 (1887): 73, 76.
45 *Transactions* 29 (1895): 34–37; *Transactions* 30 (1896): 24–25. Shortly after the turn of the century the society began campaigning vigorously for the establishment of sanitoria for "the consumptive poor"; *Wisconsin Medical Journal* 2 (1903–4): 271.
46 *Transactions* 6 (1872): 21; 8 (1874): 24; 9 (1875): 18.
47 E. A. P. Brewster, "Essay on Criminal Abortion," *Transactions* 4 (1870): 107–14. This estimate, more than twice as high as other medical estimates of the period, undoubtedly was inflated; see Mohr, *Abortion in America*, p. 81.
48 *Transactions* 2 (1868): 25–26, 52–53.
49 *Transactions* 7 (1873): 21–22; 9 (1875): 18; 10 (1876): 27.
50 "A Remedy for Evil," *Wisconsin Medical Journal* 2 (1903–4): 632–33.
51 *Wisconsin Medical Journal* 6 (1907–8): 356.
52 Holmes, "Medical Practice Sixty Yeags Ago," p. 21.
53 *Transactions* 2 (1868): 11; McNeil, "Dr. Alfred L. Castleman," p. 292. See also William S. Middleton, "The First Medical Faculty of the University of Wisconsin," *Wisconsin Medical Journal* 54 (1955): 378–85, 428–38.
54 *Transactions* 2 (1868): 77, 82; *Transactions* 3 (1869): 47; *Transactions* 4 (1870): 48.
55 *Transactions* 9 (1875): 17.
56 *Transactions* 20 (1886): 52–53; *Transactions* 21 (1887): 65; Holmes, "Medical Practice Sixty Years Ago," p. 21.
57 J. B. Whiting, "Annual Address," *Transactions* 10 (1876): 32.
58 J. K. Bartlett, "Annual Address," *Transactions* 11 (1877): 33, 38.
59 *Wisconsin Medical Journal* 6 (1907–8): 243–44.
60 *Proceedings* (1855), p. 9.
61 *Transactions* 3 (1869): 46. Stanford E. Chaillé claimed that Wisconsin was the only state society to adopt the AMA's recommendation, but another AMA report stated that the state medical societies of Maryland, New Jersey, and Kansas also approved the recommendation. See Chaillé, "State Medicine and State Medical Societies," *Transactions of the American Medical Association* 30 (1879): 355; 22 (1871): 161.
62 *Transactions* 12 (1878): 33, 36; Chaillé, "State Medicine," p. 355. For the report of the special committee, see *Transactions* 13 (1879): 256–61.
63 *Transactions* 13 (1879): 50–51, 58.
64 *Transactions* 12 (1878): 36. See also J. T. Reeve, "The Medical Profession — Its Progress and Present Position," *Transactions* 9 (1875): 27–28.
65 H. Reineking, "President's Address," *Transactions* 33 (1899): 64–65.
66 *Transactions of the American Institute of Homeopathy* (1880), p. 660; *Transactions* 14 (1880): 205–7. On homeopathy, see Thomas Lindsley Bradford, "Homeopathy in Wisconsin," in *History of Homeopathy and Its Institutions in America*, ed. William Harvey King, 4 vols. (New York: Lewis Publishing Co., 1905), 1:337–41. The minutes of the Homeopathic Medical Society of the State of Wisconsin for the years 1865–1910 and 1927–53 are in the State Historical Society of Wisconsin, Madison, Wis.

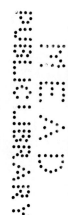

67 Alexander Wilder, *History of Medicine* (New Sharon, Maine: New England Publishing Co., 1901), p. 676. The minutes of the Wisconsin State Eclectic Medical Society for 1901 to 1934 are in the State Historical Society of Wisconsin, Madison, Wis.
68 *Transactions* 14 (1880): 46–47.
69 *Transactions* 15 (1881): 40, 48–49. During the second half of the nineteenth century the legislature adopted several laws regulating the practice of medicine, to say nothing of the dozens of bills they considered but never approved. The most important laws passed were the following.
    1867: A law stipulating that no physician or surgeon could legally enforce the collection of fees for medical services unless he possessed a diploma from an incorporated medical society or college or belonged to the state or a local medical society. *General Laws Passed by the Legislature of Wisconsin*, 1867, chap. 95, p. 89. This law, said a regular physician in 1878, "is a dead letter. It has been enforced in one or two instances, I believe, in the state; but ordinarily men collect their bills before they get to a court" (*Transactions* 12 [1878]: 36).
    1870: A law making it unlawful to practice medicine without a medical school diploma, a certificate of qualification from an incorporated medical society, or five years of experience. It did not apply to dentists, midwives, or students under a qualified preceptor. *Laws of Wisconsin*, 1870, chap. 86, pp. 141–42. Under the influence of this law, "Many a grey-headed sinner went off to take his second course of lectures. . . . The next winter the quacks flocked to Madison with any amount of money in their pockets, and they got the law repealed" (*Transactions* 13 [1879]: 52).
    1871: Repeal of the 1870 law. *Laws of Wisconsin*, 1871, chap. 144, p. 223.
    1881: "An act to prevent quacks from deceiving the people by assuming a professional title." *Laws of Wisconsin*, 1881, chap. 256, pp. 321–22.
    1882: An amendment to the 1881 law stipulating that it was not to "prevent students from practicing midwifery, nor veterinary practitioners in their special departments." Sec. 4 of the 1881 law, requiring physicians to show their diplomas or licenses on demand, was repealed. *Laws of Wisconsin*, 1882, chap. 40, p. 185.
    1897: "An act to regulate the practice of medicine and surgery in the state of Wisconsin" by establishing a board of medical examiners. *Laws of Wisconsin*, 1897, chap. 264, pp. 505–9.
70 *Transactions* 30 (1896): 32.
71 For reports of the committee on medical legislation, see *Transactions* 23 (1889): 43–44; 24 (1890): 49–50; 25 (1891): 18–21; 26 (1892): 27–28; 27 (1893): 25–26.
72 *Laws of Wisconsin*, 1897, chap. 264, pp. 505–9. Approximately 60 percent of the states had composite boards in the early twentieth century; see James G. Burrow, *Organized Medicine in the Progressive Era: The Move toward Monopoly* (Baltimore: Johns Hopkins University Press, 1977), p. 162.
73 *Transactions* 35 (1901): 20.
74 Physicians unable to surmount this barrier banded together in 1903 as the

Wisconsin Medical Union of Physicians and Surgeons to secure "liberal and just laws"; *Wisconsin Medical Journal* 2 (1903–4): 241, 512–13.

75 *Transactions* 12 (1878): 36–37.

76 *Transactions* 25 (1891): 19.

77 B. C. Brett, "President's Address," *Transactions* 28 (1894): 38. Some newspapers thought the proposed law was so narrow that it would prevent even midwives from practicing their art. Their fears were not without foundation; in 1898 the state medical society strongly recommended that the state board of medical examiners be granted power to license midwives, who, it somewhat unfairly argued, "by reason of their ignorance and filth, [were] a great danger to the life and health of the lying-in woman and her infant"; *Transactions* 31 (1897): 54; 32 (1898): 34.

78 Frank J. Campenni, *History of Dentistry* (Wisconsin State Dental Society, 1970), pp. 16, 23–28.

79 Jennifer Latham has suggested that Wisconsin's tardiness in passing a medical licensing law reflected public apathy more than anything else; "Medical Legislation in Wisconsin" (M.A. paper, University of Wisconsin–Madison, 1977).

80 *Transactions* 24 (1890): 70.

81 The State Historical Society of Wisconsin has collected the following records for the nineteenth century: Dodge County Medical Society (1894–1900), Fond du Lac County Medical Society (1868–70), Fox River Valley Medical Society (1886–1900), Lincoln County Medical Society (1893–94), North Western Wisconsin Medical Society (1879–1900), Waukesha County Medical Society (1842–1900), Winnebago County Medical Society (1865–1900), Milwaukee Medical Society (1846–81). The society's holdings for the twentieth century are even more extensive. The records of the Dane County Medical Society and the Central Wisconsin Medical Association (1851–1917) are held by the State Medical Society of Wisconsin.

82 Louis Frederick Frank, *The Medical History of Milwaukee, 1834–1914* (Milwaukee: Germania Publishing Co., 1915), pp. 132–33.

83 Minutes, Milwaukee Medical Society, May 5, 1846, State Historical Society of Wisconsin, Madison, Wis. On Milwaukee medical societies, see Frank, *Medical History of Milwaukee*, pp. 108–36; and Curtis A. Evans, "Milwaukee Medical Societies: An Eighty-Five Year Retrospect," *Wisconsin Medical Journal* 22 (1923): 245–54.

84 Minutes, Dane County Medical Society, ca. 1850–1860, State Medical Society of Wisconsin, Madison, Wis. See also William Snow Miller, "Dane County Medical Society," *Wisconsin Medical Journal* 36 (1937): 929–40; 37 (1938): 580–94; and Marianne Herriott, "Placards and Pretenders: The Dane County Medical Society in the 'Good Old Days,'" *Wisconsin Medical Journal* 75 (1976): 14–16.

85 J. M. Toner, "Statistics of Regular Medical Associations and Hospitals of the United States," *Transactions of the American Medical Association* 24 (1873): 285–333. Toner missed the Dane County Medical Society, the Milwaukee City Medical Association, and perhaps others. Earlier there existed

a Western Medical Society (*Transactions* 5 [1871]: 190) and a Walworth County Medical Society (*Transactions* 2 [1868]: 22).

86 *Transactions* 36 (1902): 430–43.

87 Fee bill of the Fox River Valley Medical Society, adopted April 24, 1894, State Historical Society of Wisconsin, Madison, Wis. See also Minutes, Dane County Medical Society, April 19, 1850, State Medical Society; and Minutes, Winnebago County Medical Society, January 11, 1866, State Historical Society.

88 Minutes, Ashland-Bayfield-Iron County Medical Society, November 14, 1932; Minutes, Brown County Medical Society, February 26, 1903, August 10, 1916, April 29, 1919, May 27, 1919, January 27, 1920, June 15, 1920, December 22, 1923 — all at the State Historical Society; and Minutes, Dane County Medical Society, September 17, 1903, July 10, 1906, September 11, 1906, October 9, 1906, State Medical Society.

89 Minutes, Winnebago County Medical Society, January 13, 1869, State Historical Society. In 1906 the Dane County Medical Society appointed a committee on dead beats.

90 Minutes, Winnebago County Medical Society, July 14, 1869, State Historical Society.

91 Minutes, Brown County Medical Society, September 25, 1919, April 6, 1920, May 4, 1920, State Historical Society.

92 Frank, *Medical History of Milwaukee*, p. 119.

93 Quoted in Evans, "Milwaukee Medical Societies," p. 246.

94 Minutes, Wisconsin Central Medical Association, July 29, 1865, State Medical Society.

95 Quoted in Davenport and Davenport, "Practicing Medicine in Madison," pp. 83–84, 86–87.

96 *Transactions* 36 (1902): 9.

97 W. H. Neilson, "President's Address," ibid., pp. 55–56.

98 Minutes, Central Wisconsin Medical Society, January 27, 1903; Minutes, Fox River Valley Medical Society, January 19, 1904, both at the State Historical Society. See also *Transactions* 36 (1902): 29.

99 Frank, *Medical History of Milwaukee*, p. 121.

100 *Wisconsin Medical Journal* 1 (1903): 279; 2 (1903–4): 41.

101 *Wisconsin Medical Journal* 2 (1903–4): 37.

102 Ibid., pp. 269, 324.

103 C. S. Sheldon, "Annual Address of the President," *Wisconsin Medical Journal* 13 (1914–15): 176; "How Wisconsin Stands," *Wisconsin Medical Journal* 14 (1915–16): 208.

104 B. C. Brett, "President's Address," *Transactions* 28 (1894): 39.

105 Minutes of the 55th Annual Session, *Transactions* 35 (1901): 20–21.

106 J. V. R. Lyman, "Annual Address of the President," *Wisconsin Medical Journal* 2 (1903–4): 153.

107 Ibid., pp. 154–55.

108 *Wisconsin Medical Journal* 4 (1905–6): 36–37, 46.

109 *Transactions of the American Institute of Homeopathy* (1906), p. 786. The

Homeopathic Medical Society of the State of Wisconsin was at its peak strength in the first decade of this century.

110 On the various activities of the state medical society, see "An Epitome of the Development and Constructive Work of the State Medical Society of Wisconsin," *Wisconsin Medical Journal* 42 (1943): 26–53.

111 On the rise of the specialty societies, see "Specialty Section," *Milwaukee Medical Times*, May 1946, pp. 73–77; John P. Mullooly, "History of the Milwaukee Internist Club: Louis M. Warfield, Founder, 1927–1971," *Milwaukee Medical Society Times* 44 (1971): 8–12; Warner S. Bump, "The Wisconsin Surgical Society: A Short History," *Wisconsin Medical Journal* 61 (1962): 593–94; J. E. Habbe, "Milwaukee's Radiologic Heritage," *Wisconsin Medical Journal* 64 (1965): 125–29; James W. Sargent, "History of Urology in Wisconsin," *Wisconsin Medical Journal* 69 (1970): 182–86. For the state medical society's reaction to the growth of these organizations, see, e.g., *Wisconsin Medical Journal* 14 (1915–16): 153–57.

112 "Workmen's Compensation," *Wisconsin Medical Journal* 15 (1916–17): 361–62.

113 T. J. Redelings, "Annual Address of the President," *Wisconsin Medical Journal* 14 (1915–16): 186.

114 *Wisconsin Medical Journal* 15 (1916–17): 283. The unanimity of opinion suggests that compulsory health insurance was not a partisan political issue among the physicians.

115 The Pennsylvania State Medical Society was the second. For a fuller discussion of these events, see Ronald L. Numbers, *Almost Persuaded: American Physicians and Compulsory Health Insurance, 1912–1920* (Baltimore: Johns Hopkins University Press, 1978).

116 *The United States of America, Appellants, vs. The American Medical Association, A Corporation . . . Appellees* (Chicago: AMA, 1941), pp. 115–17.

117 S. E. Gavin, "The President's Page," *Wisconsin Medical Journal* 36 (1937): 382.

118 "Preliminary Report of the Advisory Committee on Voluntary Sickness Insurance," *Wisconsin Medical Journal* 38 (1939): 757–809.

119 *Wisconsin Medical Journal* 48 (1949): 4.

120 *Wisconsin Medical Journal* 57 (1958): 32. The state legislature ordered the medical society to divest itself of WPS in 1977. In December 1943, the Milwaukee County Medical Society established a prepaid service plan called "Surgical Care." The threat of this plan to go statewide in 1946 prompted the state medical society to create WPS, and for years the two organizations competed aggressively with each other. James O. Kelley, "A Century of Organized Medicine," *Milwaukee Medical Times* 18 (1946): 28; *Wisconsin Medical Journal* 45 (1946): 1168–70; *Wisconsin Medical Journal* 46 (1947): 1132–33.

121 *Wisconsin Medical Journal* 53 (1954): 668.

122 J. G. Crownhart, "The Economic Status of Medicine," *Wisconsin Medical Journal* 33 (1934): 230. See also *Wisconsin Medical Journal* 45 (1946): 1176.

123 E. Minihan and T. Levi make this point in "The Political Economy of

Health Care Financing: The Foundation for Medical Care in Wisconsin,"
unpublished paper, April 1975.

124 James C. Sargent, "Shall Medicine Be Socialized?" *Wisconsin Medical Journal* 32 (1933): 562.

125 *Wisconsin Medical Journal* 54 (1955): 8. On health insurance in Wisconsin, see also A. S. Yousri, "Prepayment of Medical and Surgical Costs in Wisconsin" (Ph.D. diss., University of Wisconsin, 1956); Leon Applebaum, "A History of Voluntary Health Insurance in Wisconsin" (Ph.D. diss., University of Wisconsin 1959); Frank Sinclair, *Blue Cross in Wisconsin* (Racine: Western Printing and Lithographing Co., 1965).

126 *Wisconsin Medical Journal* 21 (1922–23): 409, 411.

127 "New Organizational Structure," *Wisconsin Medical Journal* 74 (June 1975): 52–55.

128 Charles Crownhart, "Report of the Secretary," *Wisconsin Medical Journal* 64 (1965): 374.

5 *Philip Shoemaker and Mary Van Hulle Jones*

From Infirmaries to Intensive Care: Hospitals in Wisconsin

The history of the modern hospital is a surprisingly recent story. When Wisconsin achieved statehood in 1848, the entire nation probably possessed fewer than fifty hospitals, concentrated largely in the populous cities of the Northeast.[1] These institutions generally served patients, like transients and the poor, who could not be treated at home. Physicians customarily diagnosed and treated illness, delivered babies, and even performed surgery in their patients' homes. The general hospital, as we know it today, did not appear until the late nineteenth century, when social and technological developments revolutionized the practice of medicine.

Wisconsin's earliest hospitals ministered to the homeless soldiers brought west by the United States Army. Following the War of 1812 the federal government created a network of forts in the upper Mississippi valley to protect the newly acquired frontier from Indian attack. The territory that became Wisconsin received three of these posts: Fort Howard at Green Bay (1816), Fort Crawford at Prairie du Chien (1816), and Fort Winnebago at Portage (1828).[2] Each fort included a hospital, staffed by an army surgeon and perhaps one assistant. Early inspection reports frequently describe the original wooden structures as being crowded, poorly ventilated, and dilapidated. General George Croghan, who inspected the Fort Howard hospital in 1834, reported that the building was "in such bad repair, that unless some labor be bestowed upon it, not only the poor patients, but even the medicines and stores will suffer from wet during the coming winter, as the roofs are even now not tight enough to keep out a rain."[3] The situation improved later in the 1830s, when Fort Crawford erected a stone hospital and Fort Winnebago obtained a 60-bed facility with "3 rooms and a kitchen" for the medical officer.[4]

Most soldiers admitted to fort hospitals complained of rheumatism, catarrh, ophthalmia, dysentery, diarrhea, or the ever-present "intermittent fever," better known today as malaria. Although the garrison seldom fought Indians, the hospitals reported a large number of "casualties," apparently the victims of accidental wounds.[5] In addition to caring for sick soldiers, the hospital staff also occasionally served civilians living nearby. In 1827 the Fort Howard surgeon, William Beaumont, whose experiments on the stomach of Alexis St. Martin won him international acclaim, vaccinated residents of the Fox River Valley to check a smallpox epidemic.[6] We know from Beaumont's experience at several forts that army surgeons often obtained permission to engage in private practice on the side.[7] While stationed at Fort Mackinac in Upper Michigan, Beaumont even collected fees from the county commissioners for taking care of local paupers, and on at least one occasion he admitted a private patient, the ill-fated St. Martin, into the fort hospital.[8] Unfortunately, we have not been able to determine how common this practice may have been.

By the mid-1830s the Wisconsin frontier was secure, and settlers began arriving in large numbers. The territory's population expanded tenfold during the 1840s, while Milwaukee grew from a village of 1,712 to a bustling town of over 20,000.[9] Some immigrants arrived sick and impoverished, a few suffering from smallpox or cholera. To protect the town from contagion, the Milwaukee city fathers in 1843 set up a pesthouse and ordered harbor officials to confine all immigrants showing signs of contagious disease until they recovered or died.[10] The building, an often overcrowded wooden structure "hardly large enough to accommodate a poor family of ordinary size," was run by a staff of one: a medical student.[11] The pesthouse provided neither nursing nor medical care; it existed almost solely to isolate the contagious from the healthy. If such an institution can be called a hospital, then the Milwaukee pesthouse lays claim to being Wisconsin's first nonmilitary hospital.

A more logical candidate for the honor is St. John's Infirmary, later St. Mary's Hospital, which Catholic sisters opened in Milwaukee in 1848. In the mid-1840s the bishop of Milwaukee, John Martin Henni, invited the Sisters of Charity to come from Maryland to operate a benevolent institution for the sick. On May 15, 1848, St. John's Infirmary, a two-story frame building at the corner of Jackson and Wells, opened its doors to patients of all religious and medical persuasions.[12] Although primarily for charity patients, the infirmary also provided a few select rooms for "those who are qualified to prefer them."[13]

The infirmary did not remain long at its original location. Although the sisters generally refused to accept contagious cases, neighbors feared the presence of so much sickness in their midst and pressured the infirmary into moving in 1855. The new site, on Jefferson Street, proved to be even less satisfactory. The ground was low and damp, the building decrepit, and the new neighbors just as unfriendly.[14] Finally, in 1858, the sisters accepted an offer from the city to take over the property formerly occupied by the pesthouse, which had been relocated at Wauwatosa. Where the small pesthouse had once stood, the sisters erected a three-story brick hospital capable of accommodating 55 patients in the private rooms and six wards, each of the latter equipped with a bath and water closet.[15]

As early as 1850 the sisters had set aside one ward — identified in hospital records as the Marine Hospital — to care for ailing seamen who entered the port of Milwaukee. The federal government, under the Marine Hospital Service Act of 1798, paid 50 cents per day for each sailor treated and thus provided the hospital with much of its cash income.[16] During the second half of the nineteenth century federally subsidized seamen accounted for about one-third of the hospital's census. Once on the road to recovery, they often served the hospital as waiters, laundrymen, janitors, and nurses' aides. But the sisters did not, apparently, exploit their charges. One grateful seaman described his treatment at the infirmary in 1854:

When I came here I was entirely destitute of everything even a change of Shirts or sock to put on my feet; and still continue so; but the Sisters regularly give me changes. the most esepensive Medicines is the kind that is ordered for me. It is merely to preserve for a short time Longer a lingering Carcass it is impossible to restore to health. I cannot find Language to esepress their Kindness to me and even situated as I am, they made me feel i was Favorite.[17]

Besides the sailors, the hospital had few paying patients, and thus it relied heavily on private donations and on funds paid by the county for taking care of indigent residents. Still, during its early years the hospital's finances remained precarious, with annual debts often exceeding $2,000.[18]

For decades the hospital's full-time staff consisted almost exclusively of Sisters of Charity, trained on the job. Local physicians sometimes offered their services gratuitously, and in 1848 the Milwaukee City Medical Association established a formal relationship with the hospital that provided the part-time assistance of twelve member physicians each year.[19] It was the mid-1890s, however, before St. Mary's enjoyed the services of a full-time "house physician" who actually lived in the building.

The hospital's surviving patient records reveal much about the community served by St. Mary's and the ailments from which they suffered — besides telling us a lot about the function of a general hospital in nineteenth-century Wisconsin. During the last six months of 1871, when the staff began recording such data, the average age of those entering the hospital was 25 and the typical ethnic background was German or Irish.[20] Although German-born residents made up 52 percent of the city's population and the Irish less than 8 percent, Germans accounted for only 6 percent of the hospital's patients while the Irish, perhaps attracted by the common bond of Catholicism, represented 40 percent.[21]

Until late in the century the majority of patients came for medical rather than surgical or obstetrical care and remained for an average of 24 days. In 1880, for example, 72 percent entered the hospital for medical problems: tuberculosis (19), debility (15), typhoid fever (9), pleurisy (6), alcoholism (4), insanity (4), nervousness (4), rheumatism (4), hysteria (3), intermittent fever or malaria (3), tumors (3), erysipelas (2), paralysis (2), and pneumonia (2). Most surgical patients seem to have been involved in accidents; the hospital identified six as suffering from injuries, two as having received accidental amputations, and one as being fractured. In addition, one patient had been burned and another had been scalded. Obstetrical cases are conspicuous by their absence. The hospital apparently delivered its first baby in 1875, but the number of childbirths remained negligible during the century.[22]

By 1900 the picture had changed dramatically. The mentally ill had largely disappeared into asylums, and surgery, now claiming 64 percent of the patients, had superseded medical care as the hospital's chief function. The phenomenal increase in surgery resulted primarily from the successful application of anesthesia and antisepsis (or asepsis), which allowed surgeons to explore regions of the human body hitherto forbidden. Some of the increase at St. Mary's may also have resulted from its contracts with railroad companies to care for injured workers, many of whom needed surgical assistance. Only 4.6 percent of surgical patients died in the hospital, which compared favorably with the hospital's overall mortality of approximately 6 percent for the second half of the nineteenth century.[23]

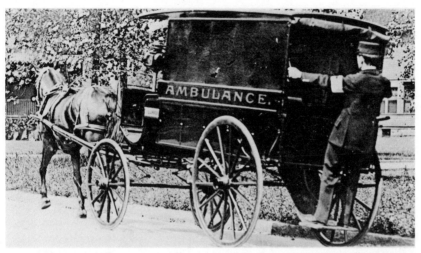

State Historical Society of Wisconsin, WHi(X3)17188

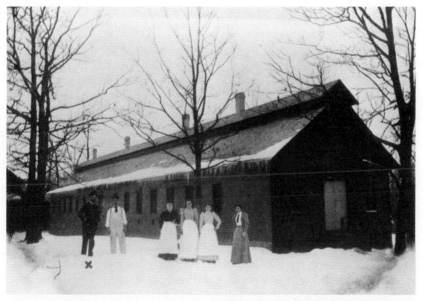

Louis Frederick Frank, *The Medical History of Milwaukee, 1834–1914*
(Milwaukee: Germania Publishing Co., 1915), p. 180

Above: In the early twentieth century horse-drawn ambulances transported Milwaukee residents to local hospitals. *Below:* In 1894 Milwaukee established a temporary smallpox hospital on the site of Downer College.

The increased popularity of surgery markedly improved the hospital's financial status, although expenditures for new surgical equipment, like the set of instruments purchased in 1895, were often substantial. Many surgical patients were neither poor nor homeless and could afford to pay the dollar-a-day charge for board, medicine, and nursing and the five-dollar fee for use of the operating room. The shift from charity to paying patients is also reflected in the hospital's practice late in the century of admitting guests who were not ill. During 1890 25 percent of those admitted to St. Mary's (excluding seamen) were either domestic servants or private nurses accompanying well-to-do patients or relatives seeking to be near their sick loved ones. On November 26, for example, a Captain Becker from New York (age 54) checked into the hospital suffering from an apparently terminal case of Bright's disease. Within a few days he was joined by an employee named Fred and two relatives, one of whom remained with the captain until his death on December 3. Like the captain, each of his visitors paid for room and board.[24]

Although hospitals like St. Mary's benefited from the popularity of surgery, some surgeons as late as the 1890s still preferred to operate in the homes of their patients, either because no hospital was available or for safety and convenience. One doctor who practiced in Manitowoc County at the close of the century recalled that

in preparing the room for surgery, water was sprinkled on the floor to settle the dust. Rubber gloves were not available, so a liberal amount of soap and water was used on the hands of the surgeon and on the site of the operation. All instruments were sterilized in the family wash boiler on the kitchen stove. I have never known of an infection following the "kitchen table operation." People were evidently immune to the germs found in their own homes.[25]

Young Dr. Adolf Gundersen of La Crosse, who arrived from Norway in 1891, similarly justified kitchen surgery on the grounds of safety. Even though he sometimes operated at St. Francis Hospital, he feared cross-contamination from other patients and complications arising from unsanitary conditions. On one occasion, for example, the old wood stove that heated the St. Francis operating room broke down and showered the entire area with soot. Often it seemed simpler and safer to visit the patient's home the day before surgery, sterilize instruments on the spot, and return the following day with an anesthetist. Gundersen reportedly performed the first appendectomy in the state in this manner.[26]

During the quarter-century following the opening of St. John's Infirmary in 1848, few other hospitals appeared in the state. When J. M. Toner in 1873 conducted his now-famous survey of hospitals in the United States, he found only 178 (including mental institutions) in the entire country and only 3 in Wisconsin: St. Mary's, the Passavant Hospital in Milwaukee, and Mendota State Hospital for the Insane near Madison.[27] He overlooked at least three others: the recently opened Northern State Hospital for the Insane in Oshkosh, the Milwaukee County Hospital, and St. Luke's Hospital in Racine. The next twenty-five years, however, witnessed a boom in hospital building. *Polk's Medical and Surgical Register* for 1900 listed 79 hospitals in Wisconsin, including 25 insane asylums but excluding numerous dispensaries, private sanatoriums, and institutional infirmaries.[28] Like St. Mary's, nearly 40 percent of the general hospitals in the state were run by Catholic sisters, a statistic that underlines the crucial role played by nuns in the history of Wisconsin medicine.[29] Although advances in medical technology, especially in surgery, contributed greatly to the proliferation of hospitals in the late nineteenth century, social changes associated with increased urbanization also seem to have prompted the establishment of general hospitals, most of which were built in urban areas.[30]

The state's few hospitals serving rural areas tended to cater to special occupational groups, like the lumberjacks of the northern counties. In the Wausau area, for example, Dr. A. W. Trevitt and his wife in 1886 opened a "ticket hospital" in a small, two-story wooden building with a capacity of 20 beds. Ticket hospitals operated in the following way: each fall an insurance agent visited the lumber camps selling ten-dollar hospital tickets to the workers, which entitled them to unlimited medical and surgical care in any participating hospital for up to one year. In addition to the Trevitts' institution, there were ticket hospitals in Eau Claire, Ashland, Marinette, and Merrill, all part of a midwestern chain that served thousands of workers by the end of the century.[31]

As *Polk's Medical and Surgical Register* indicated, nearly a third of the state's hospitals in 1900 cared for the mentally ill. Unlike the predominantly private general hospitals, the mental institutions were nearly all government supported. Although the first American asylum antedated the Revolutionary War, state mental institutions did not become popular until the second quarter of the nineteenth century, when state legislatures, prodded by Dorothea Dix and other reformers, decided to provide humane treatment for the insane. Behind the asylum movement lay the conviction that insanity, given the proper "moral treatment," was a curable disease.[32] According to the moral therapists, the mentally ill recovered best when removed from their old, immoral surroundings and placed in a family-like environment, where kindness, industry, and order prevailed.

The Wisconsin legislature began discussing the erection of an asylum in the early 1850s. After rejecting Dr. Alfred L. Castleman's profit-

ST. JOSEPH HOSPITAL

308 East Front Street,

ASHLAND, - WISCONSIN.

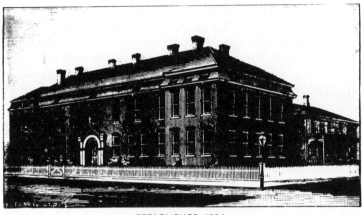

ESTABLISHED 1884.

CONDUCTED BY THE SISTERS OF POOR,

HANDMAIDS OF JESUS CHRIST.

OPEN TO ALL REGARDLESS OF RELIGIOUS BELIEF.

ANNUAL SUBSCRIPTION TICKET $7,

Which entitles the holder to Medical Attendance, Medicines and the Care of the
Sisters of this Hospital for One Year in case of Sickness or Accident.

WILL ACCOMMODATE ONE HUNDRED AND FIFTY PATIENTS.

MOTHER SUPERIOR FLAVIA, Conductress.

VISITING PHYSICIANS:

DR. G. W. HARRISON.   DR. EDWIN ELLIS.   DR. F. C. CLARK.

CONTAGIOUS DISEASES ARE EXCLUDED.

R. L. Polk and Co., *Ashland City Directory,* 1888, p. 28
(State Historical Society of Wisconsin)

In the 1880s St. Joseph Hospital in Ashland offered an early form of hospital insurance for
$7 a year.

No. 3 1 5

TICKET **$10.00**

Dated *Merrill, Wis.* 191*6*

Mr. *G. J. Synnott*

Upon payment of Ten Dollars, ($10.00) is entitled to Medicine, Admission, Medical and Surgical Treatment in the wards of DR. RAVN'S HOSPITAL, MERRILL, WIS., during one year from the date of this Certificate, in consequence of wounds, injuries, or sickness hereafter contracted, and which shall disable him from the performance of manual labor. Venereal diseases treated on this Ticket at this Hospital only.

Free Baths: Turkish, Russian, Tub and Shower.

When ordering medicine, which is sent free to any part of the country, write plainly the number of this certificate, your full name, post office and express office address. If not received promptly, notify us at once.

When badly injured or very sick, telegraph ahead, and ambulance will meet you at the train. This certificate holder agrees to comply with the rules and regulations of the various hospitals. This Certificate is not transferable, and if cancelled or altered is void.

All benefits terminate one year from above date. Excluded from this contract are:

INSANITY, CHRONIC AND CONTAGIOUS DISEASES

EXCHANGES: Marinette and Menominee Hospital, Marinette, Wis.; Jamestown City Hospital, Jamestown, N. D.; Alexian Bro's Hospital, Chicago, Ill.; Paddock Memorial Hospital Tacoma, Wash..

Agent *M. Ravn* Purchaser *G. J. Synnott*

Wisconsin lumberjacks purchased tickets like this one, issued by Dr. Ravn's Hospital in Merrill, which entitled them to hospital care in four states.

making scheme for taking care of the mentally ill (see Chapter 4, above), the legislators called in Dr. Thomas Elliott, superintendent of the Indiana state asylum, to advise them. Elliott, who subscribed to moral therapy, confidently assured the lawmakers that they could restore reason to 75 to 90 percent of the insane simply by placing them in a proper hospital environment. "The age of experiment has passed," he said. "The experience of twenty-four of your sister states . . . assures you that many thousands . . . have been restored to society and usefulness, to reason and happiness."[33]

Swayed by such prospects, the legislature voted the necessary funds, and by 1860 the state's first insane asylum was ready for occupancy. Located near Madison, on the shores of Lake Mendota, the partially completed facility initially had only 32 beds; within a year its capacity had increased to 150 and by the end of the decade to 362. The staff initially numbered 15: the superintendent (a physician), assistant physician, matron, watchman, engineer, cook, waiter, laundress, teamster, and six attendants.[34] Superintendents often complained about the low quality of attendants, who, because they had the closest contact with patients, were crucial to therapeutic success. But working conditions were far from ideal. Attendants often put in 12 to 15 hours a day, received low wages, and lived on the wards. Not surprisingly, personnel turnover was high.[35]

The Mendota institution grew rapidly as the state's insane, formerly shut away in jails, poorhouses, and attics, streamed into the facility. By 1870 it could accommodate no more patients; so the legislature voted to build a second state asylum, in Oshkosh, on the shores of Lake Winnebago. (Scenic locations provided the serenity necessary for effective moral treatment.) This, too, filled almost immediately. Of the 205 patients who entered the Winnebago hospital during its first year, 34 were over 50 years of age and 4 were in their eighties.[36] Over half had been insane all their lives. The ethnic distribution of the 89 patients admitted to Mendota in 1860 reflected the state's population: 49 were American-born, 20 German-born, 11 Irish-born, and 9 came from other countries.[37]

By the late 1870s some observers were expressing concern that the two state institutions, with hundreds of patients, were too large to be effective, that their function had changed from a curative to a custodial one. To remedy the situation, Dr. Thomas Reed, one-time speaker of the state assembly, proposed a system of small county asylums, "equal in all essential respects, and far better in some," than the state hospitals.[38] Within a few years Reed had convinced his colleagues, and in 1881 the state undertook a program, unprecedented in the United States, whereby it promised to pay for the care of indigent patients in county asylums. By 1900 there were 24 such institutions.[39]

Unfortunately, the high expectations of mid-century were never realized: the majority of those who entered the asylums never recovered. After three years of operation, the Mendota superintendent reported a recovery rate of only 15 percent. When Dr. Charles R. Bardeen surveyed Wisconsin's asylums in 1923, he found that only 2 percent of their patients had been cured.[40]

During the twentieth century Wisconsin led all states but New York, with a much larger population, in number of mental institutions.[41] Following the Second World War the appearance of tranquilizers and an emphasis on short-term and out-patient care led to the establishment of psychiatric units in several large urban hospitals and brought about a decline in the number of mental hospitals[42] (see Figure 5.1). The surviving institutions, however, continued to play a vital role in meeting the needs of the mentally ill.

The state's experience with asylums for the mentally ill suggested a model for dealing with an even more pressing health problem: tuberculosis.[43] At the turn of the century tuberculosis ranked first among causes of death in the state[44] and second to influenza-pneumonia nationwide.[45]

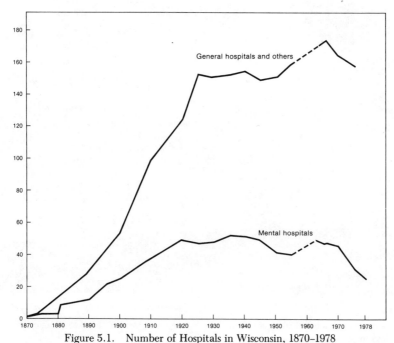

Figure 5.1.   Number of Hospitals in Wisconsin, 1870–1978

Sources: *Transactions of the American Medical Association* 24 (1873): 332; *Polk's Medical Register* for 1890, 1900, and 1910; "Hospital Service in the United States," *Journal of the American Medical Association* for the years 1926–1951; "Hospital Statistics," *Hospitals*, guide issues for 1956 and 1961; *American Medical Directory*, 7th ed. (Chicago: American Medical Association, 1921), pp. 1584–87; *General Hospitals, Mental Hospitals, Tuberculosis Hospitals and Related Institutions Licensed or Approved in Wisconsin* (Madison: Wisconsin State Board of Health, 1963, 1965, and 1966); annual publications of *Directory of General and Special Hospitals in Wisconsin*, 1970–1979 (Madison: Department of Health and Social Services); Bernett O. Odegard and George M. Keith, *A History of the State Board of Control of Wisconsin and State Institutions, 1849–1939* (Madison: State Board of Control, n.d.), pp. 160, 163. Broken lines indicate unconfirmed sources.

In 1875 a private physician in Asheville, North Carolina, opened the first private sanatorium for the tubercular, and soon similar institutions began appearing elsewhere.[46]

Early in the twentieth century, after the University of Wisconsin School of Agriculture succeeded in controlling and to some extent eradicating tuberculosis in cattle, citizens hoping to do the same for humans began demanding a state sanatorium for people suffering from the disease. General hospitals, they argued, should no longer bear the responsibility of isolating and caring for tubercular patients. After several years of debate the legislature in 1905 finally passed an act calling for the creation of a state sanatorium.[47] This institution, built on large tract

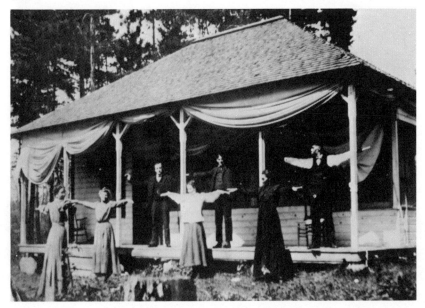

Tuberculosis patients at the Evergreen Park Cottage Sanatorium in Lake Nebagamon exercised in the open air.

two miles from the village of Wales in Waukesha County, opened in the fall of 1907. By the following spring it was filled beyond its 60-bed capacity.[48]

Perhaps inspired by the government's activity, private groups of physicians also began establishing special tuberculosis hospitals: the River Pines Sanatorium at Stevens Point and the Blue Mound Sanatorium near Milwaukee. Together with the state sanatorium, these institutions provided 132 beds — approximately one bed for every 18 deaths from tuberculosis in the state — and placed Wisconsin among the nation's leaders in providing for the victims of the so-called white plague.[49]

Despite the availability of these institutions, the need for additional facilities, especially in the northern and western parts of the state, soon became clear. Thus in 1911 the legislature approved a plan to create a system of county sanatoriums similar to the network of insane asylums.[50] By 1930 the number of tuberculosis hospitals in Wisconsin reached its maximum of 22 (see Figure 5.2).[51] In addition, the state ran a 526-acre camp and farm (established in 1913) at Little Lake Tomahawk in Oneida County to provide care for persons recovering from tuberculosis. Working out in the fresh air, many of these patients gradually recovered sufficient strength to return to their normal occupations.[52]

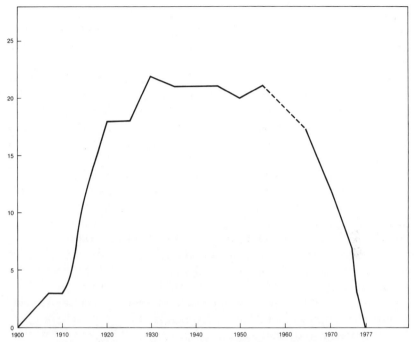

Figure 5.2.   Number of Tuberculosis Hospitals in Wisconsin, 1900–1977
Sources: Bernett O. Odegard and George M. Keith, *A History of the State Board of Control of Wisconsin and State Institutions, 1849–1939* (Madison: State Board of Control, n.d.), pp. 135–53; "Hospital Service in the United States," *Journal of the American Medical Association* for the years 1926–1951; "Hospital Statistics," *Hospitals*, guide issues for 1956 and 1961; *American Medical Directory*, 7th ed. (Chicago: American Medical Association, 1921), pp. 1584–87; *General Hospitals, Mental Hospitals, Tuberculosis Hospitals and Related Institutions Licensed or Approved in Wisconsin*, (Madison: Wisconsin State Board of Health, 1963, 1965, and 1966); annual publications of *Directory of General and Special Hospitals in Wisconsin*, 1970–1979.

Until after the Second World War, when streptomycin was introduced, medicine had little to offer sufferers of tuberculosis besides rest, fresh air, and a proper diet. (Surgery was sometimes employed to collapse an affected lung, allowing it to rest and theoretically speeding up recovery;[53] but the value of this procedure is uncertain.) Sanatoriums did, however, isolate some contagious carriers from the rest of society and thus may have contributed a little to lowering the death rate from tuberculosis, which declined rapidly during the first half of the twentieth century.[54] By 1955 the campaign against tuberculosis had proven so successful that the legislature voted to permit the conversion of county sanatoriums into county homes for the aged and chronically ill. Two years later the state shut down its sanatorium at Wales and its rehabilitation camp at Little Lake Tomahawk.[55] By the late 1970s, although a few beds for tuberculosis patients were available in general and rehabilitation hospitals, not a single tuberculosis hospital remained in the state.[56]

While the number of mental and tuberculosis hospitals rose and fell during the twentieth century, the capacity of general hospitals steadily expanded, though the total declined in the 1960s. Between 1900 and 1975 the number of general hospitals in Wisconsin tripled, from 53 to 159 (see Figure 5.1, above), and the number of beds in such institutions increased nearly sevenfold, from approximately 3,500 to 23,500.[57] Although many of the new hospitals had no religious connection, church-related institutions continued to provide a substantial amount of hospital care in the state. During the half-century between the 1920s and 1970s their share of hospital beds rose from 23 to 35 percent, even though the number of such institutions declined from 60 to 50.[58]

The story of Madison General Hospital tells much about the history of twentieth-century hospitals, as did St. Mary's in Milwaukee for the nineteenth century. In 1898 a group of Madison's most prominent citizens incorporated themselves as the Madison General Hospital Association for the purpose of establishing a general public hospital to be operated "according to the most approved principles of hygiene."[59] At that time the city's meager hospital facilities consisted of the state mental hospital at Mendota, a small municipal isolation hospital, Mrs. Mary Hayes's private hospital for ten patients, which she operated out of a house on East Doty Street,[60] and the city jail, which took care of charity cases.[61] In 1900, after a brief period of assisting Mrs. Hayes, the association took over the Hayes Hospital and rented a double house with accommodations for 16 patients.[62] But the association members still were not satisfied. They felt that Madison, home of the state university, the capital, and a busy railroad center serving a population of about 20,000, deserved a large, modern, well-managed hospital.[63] With $15,000 from the city and a matching sum raised by public subscription and donations, they succeeded in building a new facility.[64]

The new 30-bed Madison General Hospital opened in October 1903, welcoming patients of all social classes. In addition to its nine private rooms and five wards, it featured operating and anesthetizing rooms and quarters for nurses on the third floor.[65] By the close of its second year in operation, the need for a much larger building was already apparent.[66] The demand for private rooms far exceeded the supply, and many medical and obstetrical patients had to be cared for at home in order to provide beds for surgical patients, who received preferential treatment.[67]

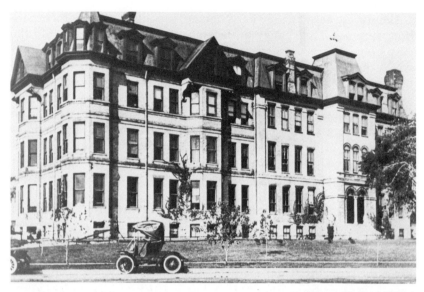

Courtesy of St. Mary's Hospital

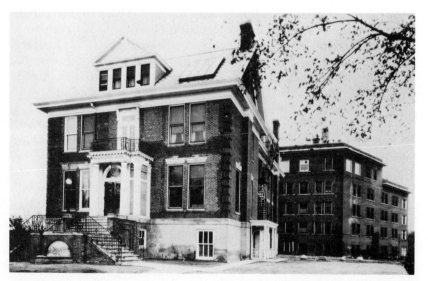

State Historical Society of Wisconsin, WHi(X3)21498

Above: St. Mary's Hospital in Milwaukee about 1905. *Below:* Madison General Hospital about 1920.

Despite the hospital's obvious popularity, additional funds for expansion were not immediately forthcoming.[68] However, late in 1910 the City Council turned over to the association title to part of the land on which the hospital stood, thus making it possible for the association to borrow a portion of the money needed to build an addition.[69] The remainder came from public subscriptions and donations, some of which had interesting strings attached. Dr. Reginald Jackson paid for the cost of constructing a private operating room — on condition that he have exclusive use of it for as long as he practiced surgery. And T. E. Brittingham gave $5,000 in return for a promise that the hospital would at all times maintain a free bed for needy students from the University of Wisconsin.[70]

As a result of such fund raising, Madison General early in 1912 moved into a new fireproof building, designed with the most up-to-date features: monolithic floors, solariums, sun porches, diet kitchens, dressing, delivery, and operating rooms, and isolation, hydrotherapeutic, and X-ray departments. There were no frills, however; the association had consciously sacrificed ornaments and elaborate finishes in order to provide the real essentials.[71]

By 1915 three other hospitals had appeared in the city: the Madison Sanitarium, a 40-bed water cure and general hospital operated since 1903 by the Seventh-day Adventists; St. Mary's, a Catholic hospital opened in 1912; and a small maternity hospital.[72] Nevertheless, Madison General found expansion a recurring necessity as it struggled to meet the needs of an ever-growing city, destined to become second largest in the state by mid-century. From a bed capacity of slightly over 100 in the late 1910s, Madison General grew to more than 125 beds in 1921, 175 in 1929, 400 in 1954, and about 480 in 1978.[73]

As the hospital expanded, so inevitably did its staff. The original double house with 16 beds had been staffed by one superintendent, three nurses, a cook, laundress, janitor, and two young women. There was no medical staff, although any reputable physician or surgeon could use the hospital's facilities.[74] The new building that opened in 1903 allowed for the addition of more than a dozen student nurses and the hospital's first physician intern, appointed in 1906.[75] Before long the institution had grown so large that the association appointed a medical staff to formulate rules for surgical and medical practice in the hospital (action that won a Class A rating from the American College of Surgeons[76]) and created two superintendencies, one for the hospital, the other for nurses.[77] By mid-century the medical staff included 133 physicians. In addition, the hospital now supported 5 residents, 3 interns, 62 nurses,

92 student nurses, 97 orderlies and attendants, plus approximately 200 other employees, including anesthetists, X-ray technicians, medical technicians, dietitians, and a pharmacist.[78]

The function of the hospital also changed substantially during this period, although surgery remained its most important activity (see Figure 5.3). During the early years appendectomies ranked first among the hospital's surgical operations[79] — despite a widespread suspicion that appendicitis was nothing but a money-making invention of surgeons.[80] Early-twentieth-century surgeons at Madison General also set broken bones, repaired wounds, amputated limbs, and performed such relatively complex procedures as hernia repairs and gall bladder operations, the latter made reasonably safe by improvements in anesthetics and aseptic techniques.[81] Such improvements may also have contributed to the increased number of obstetrical cases at Madison General, as word spread that hospital deliveries were safer, less painful, and even less expensive than those at home.[82] By the early 1950s home births in Wisconsin had plummeted to 1 percent, down from 62 percent just two decades earlier.[83]

From the beginning, surgical cases outnumbered both medical and obstetrical cases at Madison General (Figure 5.3). At first medical patients were admitted only when space permitted, with "positively" no contagious cases allowed.[84] This ban remained in effect until the great influenza epidemic of 1918, when the hospital accepted 328 influenza cases between October and December alone.[85] In the late 1920s the hospital inaugurated a new service for medical patients, based on "the clinic idea." Under this system ambulatory patients could take advantage of the institution's diagnostic facilities without checking into the hospital. This saved both time and money.[86] Other developments reflected the growing specialization of medicine. By the late 1950s Madison General boasted 16 different medical services, ranging from orthopedics and urology to psychiatry and neurosurgery,[87] and within two decades these had expanded to cover scores of medical specialties and subspecialties, each utilizing expensive and sophisticated equipment. Of course, none of this came without a price.

Perhaps no aspect of hospitalization in the twentieth century attracted more attention than the spectacular rise in costs. When Madison General opened its new building in 1903, patients could choose between wards at $5 to $10 per week and private rooms for $10 to $25 per week, with food, medical supplies, and nursing care included. Operating-room fees ($5) and physician and surgeon charges were extra. The hospital accepted charity patients sent by the city physician or by private

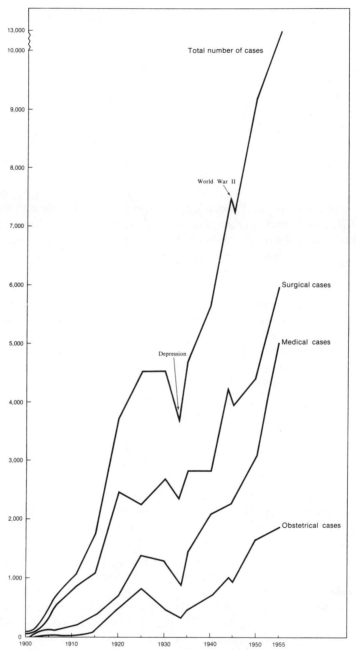

Figure 5.3.   Number of Cases, 1900–1955, Madison General Hospital
Source: Annual Reports of Madison General Hospital, 1901–1955.

practitioners who waived their own fees; however, no free patients could remain in the hospital longer than six weeks except by special order of the association's executive committee.[88]

Madison General succeeded in keeping costs relatively low during its early years not only by offering a limited range of services, but also by training nurses and doctors, who provided inexpensive professional help in exchange for little more than food, a bed, and the experience. The rise of hospital nursing schools accompanied the late-nineteenth-century boom in hospital construction. Inspired by the achievements of Florence Nightingale in England and by the need to provide low-cost medical care, American hospitals in 1873 began to offer apprenticeship training for young women wanting to become nurses. By 1900 there were 432 such schools,[89] many of them affiliated with tiny hospitals that "trained" two or three nurses a year with little regard for educational standards. Despite the exploitative nature of these institutions, students flocked to them, largely, it seems, because American women had few other career choices besides teaching open to them.[90]

The nursing school at Madison General began in 1902, only eight years after St. Mary's had opened its school and 14 years after the founding of the state's first nursing schools.[91] Madison General required candidates for admission to be between 21 and 31 years of age, to possess a high school diploma or equivalent, to present letters of reference testifying to their physical and moral fitness, to offer proof of vaccination — and to display "teeth in perfect order." The so-called curriculum, typical of such schools, called for two years of training until 1914, after which three years were required. Students customarily worked 12-hour shifts, from seven to seven, with two hours off each weekday (when possible), a free afternoon once a week, and a two-week vacation each year. In return for their services, students received room and board and — after a one-month probationary period — $6 a month for the purchase of uniforms and books.[92]

Physician interns fared little better. After 1915 they needed the one-year experience in a hospital in order to obtain a license to practice medicine in the state, and hospitals inevitably took advantage of the situation to tap a second source of cheap labor.[93] The common view of the intern can be seen in the advice one speaker gave to the Wisconsin Hospital Association on how to attract interns. Referring to these young doctors as the "goats" of the staff, he advised hospital administrators not to treat them like janitors or orderlies, but to give them adequate quarters, good food, and ample recreation.[94]

Madison General, which appointed its first intern in 1906, required interns to sign a one-year contract, binding the physician to full-time service and to scrupulous observance of all the hospital's rules and regulations. These called for interns to live in the hospital, to be on call at all times, to engage in no work outside the hospital, and to abstain from talking with nurses while on duty except when necessary in the course of work. The intern's responsibilities included examining all patients admitted to the hospital, taking careful case histories, making thorough physical and clinical examinations, and keeping accurate records of each case.[95] After 1921 the hospital paid interns $25 a month.[96]

With the advent of licensing regulations that imposed educational requirements on nursing schools[97] and with increased competition among hospitals for interns and residents, the two traditional sources of inexpensive professional help began drying up. But this development constituted only a small part of the growing financial problem plaguing hospitals in the twentieth century. Already by 1913, when private rooms at Madison General went for $2.50 to $4.00 a day, the president of the association expressed concern that few residents could afford even $3.00 a day for hospital care.[98] During the next decade the Wisconsin Hospital Association became increasingly troubled by the inability of middle-class citizens to pay for hospital care.[99] As Dr. W. H. Smith told the American Medical Association in 1921: "The hospitals provide for the poor and well-to-do, but make no special provision for that large class of persons of moderate means."[100]

The Great Depression drove the nation's hospitals into even deeper financial difficulty. Revenue from patients fell precipitously and charity loads almost quadrupled.[101] Although Madison General weathered the first year or so of depression fairly well, by 1931 it was feeling the economic pinch. Between 1930 and 1933 the number of patients seeking admission dropped from 4,530 to 3,661, while the charity load more than doubled.[102] To make matters worse, the Community Chest reduced its subsidy to the hospital, forcing it to rely even more heavily on gifts, bequests, and its shrinking income from endowments.[103]

In response to the disastrous economic effects of the depression, a number of American hospitals began experimenting with prepayment plans, whereby members received complete hospital care in return for a fixed monthly charge. The success of these early plans led to the creation of Blue Cross hospitalization insurance.[104] Blue Cross did not come to Wisconsin until 1939, too late to assist with the depression, but just in time to help cope with the rapidly rising costs of hospitalization, which doubled between 1942 and 1952.[105] As an officer of the Madison General Hospital Association reported in 1941, group insurance plans covering company employees, city workers, and others virtually eliminated unpaid hospital bills for those enrolled.[106] Such insurance plans proved so popular that by the early 1960s nearly three-fourths of all American families had at least partial coverage.[107] The passage of Medicare and Medicaid legislation in 1965 extended this protection to millions of the elderly and the poor, who often could not afford private insurance. By 1968 Madison General took in only 25 percent of its gross revenue directly from patients; the remainder came from insurance, 50 percent from private carriers like Blue Cross, and 25 percent from Medicare and Medicaid payments.[108] At last, through health insurance, the hospital had discovered a relatively stable way of financing its ever-more-expensive activities.

By the 1970s the general hospital had come to occupy a central place in providing health care to the citizens of Wisconsin. Only a century before, the state's few hospitals had offered limited care to a relative handful of poor Milwaukeeans and transients, while virtually all physicians continued to diagnose and treat their patients at home. As late as 1910 almost half of the counties in the state still had no general hospital; fifty years later the number had declined to three (see Table 5.1). Following the Second World War and the implementation of the Hill-Burton Program providing federal funds for the construction of hospitals, high-quality institutions became common throughout the state, and medical care actually grew *less* centralized.[109] Given excellent hospital facilities in cities like La Crosse, Marshfield, and Eau Claire, physicians began spreading out across the state rather than congregating in Milwaukee and Madison.[110] To what extent the citizens of Wisconsin benefited from these developments remains to be seen.

Table 5.1. Number of Wisconsin Counties with Specified Ratios of Population to Hospital Beds, by Decade, 1910–1960[a]

Population–Hospital Bed Ratio	Number of Counties					
	1910	*1920*	*1930*	*1940*	*1950*	*1960*
200 or less	4	5	6	5	5	19
201–400	8	11	18	23	36	32
401–600	4	7	10	20	15	12
601 or more	21	20	19	12	9	3
No general hospital	32	26	16	9	4	3
Total	69	69	69	69	69	69

Source: Gordon Bultena, *The Changing Distribution and Adequacy of Medical, Dental, and Hospital Services in Rural and Urban Communities in Wisconsin, 1910–1960* (Madison: Department of Rural Sociology bulletin, College of Agriculture, University of Wisconsin, May, 1966), p. 18.
[a]The data are for general hospitals only and do not include beds in specialized hospitals such as tuberculosis sanatoriums or in nursing homes.

Notes

The authors wish to thank Ronald L. Numbers, who supervised the writing of this chapter; Sister Priscilla Grimes, Administrator of St. Mary's Hospital in Milwaukee, and Peter Hanson, Director of Community Relations, who graciously made available the records of St. Mary's Hospital; the Public Relations Department of the Madison General Hospital; the Wisconsin Hospital Association; and the librarians of the Wisconsin State Historical Society. Mr. Shoemaker also wishes to acknowledge the assistance of his wife, Janet.

1 J. M. Toner, "Statistics of Regular Medical Associations and Hospitals of the United States," *Transactions of the American Medical Association* 24 (1873): 314. Toner listed 49 hospitals established before 1850.

2 For more information, see Charles R. Bardeen's series of articles, "Hospitals in Wisconsin; A Historical Survey, 1816–1925," *Wisconsin Medical Journal* 24 (1925); and Peter L. Scanlan, "Points of Prairie du Chien History," undated, Peter L. Scanlan Papers, State Historical Society of Wisconsin, Madison, Wis.

3 George Croghan, "Report of an Inspection of the United States Forces and Military Posts," Fort Howard, August 2, 1834, from a photocopy in "Inspection Reports," Vol. 5 (1830–36), Archives Division, State Historical Society of Wisconsin, Madison, Wis.

4 Croghan, "Report of an Inspection," Fort Winnebago, August 7, 1834.

5 Croghan, "Report of an Inspection," Fort Howard, August 2, 1834.

6 William Miller, "Beaumont, The Man," Peter L. Scanlan Papers, State Historical Society of Wisconsin, Madison, Wis.

7 Jesse S. Myer, *Life and Letters of Dr. William Beaumont* (St. Louis: C. V. Mosby Co., 1939), pp. 82, 239.

8 Minutes, Michilimackinac County Commissioners, December 3, 1821–January 31, 1859, microfilm copy from the State of Michigan Department of Natural Resources, Mackinac Island State Park Commission.

9 Bayrd Still, *Milwaukee: The History of a City* (Madison: State Historical Society, 1948), p. 570.

10 Peter Leo Johnson, *Daughters of Charity in Milwaukee, 1846–1946* (Milwaukee: Daughters of Charity, 1946), p. 30.

11 Ibid., pp. 30–31.

12 Ibid., p. 38.

13 Quoted ibid.

14 Ibid., pp. 62, 68.

15 Ibid., p. 80.

16 Ibid., p. 90.

17 Patrick Kelley to Margaret Gallagher, Milwaukee, July 24, 1854, Archives, St. Mary's Hospital, Milwaukee, Wis.

18 Johnson, *Daughters of Charity*, pp. 90–91.

19 Ibid., p. 39.

20 "List of Patients, 1859–1900," Archives, St. Mary's Hospital, Milwaukee, Wis.

21 Ibid.
22 Ibid. The average length of hospitalization is computed from data found in the patient records. In 1875 the sisters reported three cases of "confinement," along with the names of the children born.
23 Ibid. In 1900 hospital physicians performed 428 operations, 18 of which resulted in the death of the patient.
24 Ibid., pp. 104–5.
25 F. W. Hammond, "Seventy Years in the Practice of Medicine," Manitowoc County Historical Society, *Occupational Monograph 6*, 1968 series, p. 5.
26 Berit H. Midelfort, "Adolf Gundersen: The Physician and His Effect upon the Medical Community in and around La Crosse," undated manuscript, courtesy of the author.
27 Toner, "Medical Associations and Hospitals," p. 314.
28 *Polk's Medical and Surgical Register of the United States and Canada* (Chicago: R. L. Polk and Co., 1900), pp. 1809–13.
29 Benjamin Blied, "Wisconsin's Catholic Hospitals," *The Salesianum* 43 (1948): 10–19.
30 Morris J. Vogel, "Boston's Hospitals, 1870–1930: A Social History" (Ph.D. diss., University of Chicago, 1974), pp. 200–244.
31 S. M. E. Smith, "Sketch of Medical Practice and Hospitals in the Wausau Area," undated, Archives Division, State Historical Society of Wisconsin, Madison, Wis.
32 Gerald Grob, *Mental Institutions in America: Social Policy to 1875* (New York: The Free Press, 1973), pp. 35, 182–86.
33 Thomas Elliott, *An Address to the Legislature, in Behalf of the Insane of the State of Wisconsin* (Madison: Calkins and Proudfit, 1856), p. 11, bound in Wisconsin State Hospital for the Insane, *Reports*, Vol. 1, pp. 1854–67.
34 "Superintendent's Report," in the *Annual Report of the Board of Trustees, of the Wisconsin State Hospital for the Insane* (Madison: James Ross, State Printer, 1860), pp. 30–31, bound in Wisconsin State Hospital for the Insane, *Reports*, Vol. 1.
35 Julaine Farrow, *Winnebago State Hospital, 1873–1973* (Madison: State Historical Society, 1973), pp. 128–38. In 1879, for example, only 17 of the 95 employees remained on the job for more than one year.
36 Ibid., p. 6.
37 "Superintendent's Report," in *Annual Report, Board of Trustees*, p. 26.
38 Thomas Reed, "Journal," undated, Archives Division, State Historical Society of Wisconsin, Madison, Wis.
39 *Polk's Medical Register*, 1900, pp. 1809–13.
40 Bardeen, "Hospitals in Wisconsin," p. xxviii.
41 "Hospital Service in the United States," *Journal of the American Medical Association* 90 (1928): 913. For annual statistics, see "Hospital Service in the United States," contained in each volume of the *Journal* from 1928 to 1953; bound in a separate volume in the Middleton Medical Library at the University of Wisconsin–Madison.

42 *Wisconsin State Plan for Hospital and Medical Facilities, 1959–1960* (Madison: Wisconsin Board of Health, n.d.), p. 158.

43 Bernett O. Odegard and George M. Keith, *A History of the State Board of Control of Wisconsin and State Institutions, 1849–1939* (Madison: State Board of Control, n.d.), p. 150.

44 *Twentieth Report of the State Board of Health of Wisconsin* (Madison, 1905), p. 144.

45 Judith Walzer Leavitt and Ronald L. Numbers, eds., *Sickness and Health in America: Readings in the History of Medicine and Public Health* (Madison: University of Wisconsin Press, 1978), p. 7.

46 Odegard and Keith, *History of the State Board of Control*, p. 136.

47 Ibid., p. 138.

48 Ibid., pp. 138–39.

49 Ibid., p. 149.

50 Ibid., p. 150.

51 "Hospital Service in the United States," *Journal of the American Medical Association* 96 (1931): 1012.

52 Odegard and Keith, *History of the State Board of Control*, p. 147.

53 Albert G. Bower and Edith B. Pilant, *Communicable Diseases for Nurses*, 6th ed. (Philadelphia: W. B. Saunders Co., 1949), pp. 348–51.

54 Odegard and Keith, *History of the State Board of Control*, p. 152. In the thirty years following the opening of the sanatorium at Wales, the death rate from tuberculosis per hundred thousand population decreased from 109.3 in 1908 to 33.1 in 1937.

55 *Wisconsin State Plan for Hospital and Medical Facilities, 1959–1960*, p. 149.

56 *General and Special Hospitals in Wisconsin* (Madison: Bureau of Quality Compliance, Division of Health, Department of Health and Social Services, 1978), facing p. 1.

57 For 1900 figures, see *Polk's Medical Register*, 1900, pp. 1810–13. For 1975 figures, see *Directory of General and Special Hospitals in Wisconsin* (Madison: Division of Health, Department of Health and Social Services, 1975). These figures include general hospitals and those special hospitals, such as maternity and emergency hospitals, which are often departments of general hospitals. They exclude tuberculosis and mental hospitals. The 1900 and 1910 figures also exclude the "sanitariums," listed separately in *Polk's Register*, 1900, pp. 1810–13, and *Polk's Medical Register*, 1910 (Detroit: R. L. Polk and Co., 1910), pp. 1941–45, since these were primarily for nervous or mental disorders and rest cures. The number of general hospitals remained fairly consistent after 1925 (around 150), but their bed capacity steadily grew larger.

58 For 1927 figures, see "Hospital Service in the United States," *Journal of the American Medical Association* 90 (1928): 915. For 1970's figures, see *Directory of General and Special Hospitals in Wisconsin* (Madison: Division of Health, Department of Health and Social Services, 1976).

59 *Second Annual Report of the Madison General Hospital and Training*

School for Nurses (Madison: Madison General Hoapital, 1902), p. 26. All Madison General Hospital reports cited in this chapter were published by Madison General Hospital, Madison, Wis.

60 *Polk's Medical Register,* 1900, pp. 1810–13. For contagious hospitals, see *Polk's Medical Register* for 1910, p. 1942.

61 Siegrid Fredrickson, "The Contribution of the Spanish Influenza Pandemic of 1918–1919 to the Advancement of Hospital Care in Madison, Wisconsin," manuscript, 1978, p. 2., courtesy of the author. On nineteenth-century hospitals in Madison, see "Early Hospitals," *Wisconsin State Journal,* January 6, 1898, p. 1. We wish to thank Richard C. Kosmer, Jr., for bringing this to our attention.

62 *Annual Report, Madison General Hospital Association* (1901), pp. 4–5.

63 *Fourth Annual Report of the Madison General Hospital and Training School for Nurses* (1904), p. 11.

64 *Second Annual Report of the Madison General Hospital,* pp. 7–9.

65 *Fourth Annual Report of the Madison General Hospital,* pp. 6, 11, 14, 16, 30, 44.

66 *Fifth Annual Report of the Madison General Hospital and Training School for Nurses* (1905), p. 11.

67 *Eighth Annual Report of the Madison General Hospital and Training School for Nurses* (1908), p. 13.

68 *Eleventh Annual Report of the Madison General Hospital and Training School for Nurses* (1911), pp. 10–11.

69 Ibid., pp. 14–15. For original financial arrangements with the City of Madison, see pp. 9–10.

70 *Twelfth Annual Report of the Madison General Hospital and Training School for Nurses* (1912), p. 15.

71 *Thirteenth Annual Report of the Madison General Hospital and Training School for Nurses* (1913), p. 4.

72 C. P. Farnsworth, "The Madison (Wis.) Sanitarium," *Advent Review and Sabbath Herald* 82 (1905): 19–20; *Polk's Medical Register, 1917* (Detroit: R. L. Polk and Co., 1917), pp. 1570–75. An annex to the Madison Sanitarium accommodated 25 patients, giving it a total capacity of over 60 beds.

73 *Eighteenth and Nineteenth Annual Reports of the Madison General Hospital and Training School for Nurses* (1919), p. 10; *Twentieth, Twenty-First and Twenty-Second Annual Reports of the Madison General Hospital and Training School for Nurses* (1922), p. 13; *Thirtieth Annual Report of the Madison General Hospital and School of Nursing* (1930), p. 20; *Fifty-Fifth Annual Report of the Madison General Hospital* (1955), p. 8; *General and Special Hospitals in Wisconsin* (Madison: Division of Health, Department of Health and Social Services, 1979).

74 *Second Annual Report of the Madison General Hospital,* pp. 3, 5, 13–16.

75 *Sixth Annual Report of the Madison General Hospital and Training School for Nurses* (1906), p. 6.

76 *Twentieth, Twenty-First and Twenty-Second Annual Reports of the Madison General Hospital,* pp. 93, 94, 227, 228. In 1910 a medical board had

been appointed whose members acted in an advisory capacity to the Executive Committee of the Hospital Association. This was not a medical staff for the hospital. The members of the medical board had charge of all charity patients, as well as those who applied directly to the hospital for treatment. For membership and rules regulating this board, see the *Tenth Annual Report of the Madison General Hospital and Training School for Nurses* (1910), pp. 5, 43. Also see *Twelfth Annual Report of the Madison General Hospital*, pp. 7, 59.

77 *Eighth Annual Report of the Madison General Hospital*, pp. 3, 13, 15.

78 *Fifty-First Annual Report of the Madison General Hospital* (1951), p. 9d.

79 See the annual reports of Madison General Hospital for the years 1903 through 1908.

80 Taped interview with Louis Van Hulle, September 29, 1978.

81 See the annual reports of Madison General Hospital for the years 1902 through 1929.

82 *Sixteenth Annual Report of the Madison General Hospital and Training School for Nurses* (1916), p. 15.

83 Louis Block, *Hospital Trends* (Chicago: Hospital Topics, 1956), p. 46.

84 *Third Annual Report of the Madison General Hospital and Training School for Nurses* (1903), p. 5.

85 *Eighteenth and Nineteenth Annual Reports of the Madison General Hospital*, p. 78. See also Fredrickson, "The Contribution of the Spanish Influenza Pandemic," p. 6.

86 *Twenty-Eighth Annual Report of the Madison General Hospital and School of Nursing* (1928), p. 24.

87 *Fifty-Eighth Annual Report of the Madison General Hospital* (1958), p. 21. A physical therapy department had been established in 1926 (*Twenty-Seventh Annual Report of the Madison General Hospital and School of Nursing* [1927], p. 45). A social service department was added in 1929 (*Thirtieth Annual Report of the Madison General Hospital*, p. 24). By 1957 there was also an occupational therapy department (*Fifty-Eighth Annual Report of the Madison General Hospital*, p. 27).

88 *Fourth Annual Report of the Madison General Hospital*, pp. 6–7.

89 Richard Harrison Shryock, "Nursing Emerges as a Profession: The American Experience," in Leavitt and Numbers, eds., *Sickness and Health in America*, p. 205.

90 Signe Cooper, "Early Schools of Nursing in Wisconsin," manuscript, 1978, pp. 11, 12, courtesy of the author.

91 *Fifteenth Annual Report of the Madison General Hospital and Training School for Nurses* (1915), p. 9; Carol Moroder Oberbreckling, ed., *Saint Mary's School of Nursing, formerly Saint Mary's Training School for Nurses, 1894–1969* (Milwaukee, Wis.: Alumnae Association, St. Mary's School of Nursing, 1969), p. 18; Cooper, "Early Schools of Nursing," p. 3.

92 *Seventh Annual Report of the Madison General Hospital and Training School for Nurses* (1907), p. 15; *Fifteenth Annual Report of the Madison*

General Hospital, pp. 9–10; *Seventh Annual Report of the Madison General Hospital*, pp. 15–16.

93 *Wisconsin Medical Journal* 14 (1915–16): 160, 164. By 1915 twenty-one states required an internship before the medical graduate could take the state board examination for licensure.

94 Minutes of the Annual Meeting of the Wisconsin Hospital Association, May 18, 1923, Archives, Wisconsin Hospital Association, Madison, Wis.

95 *Eighteenth and Nineteenth Annual Reports of the Madison General Hospital*, pp. 126–27.

96 *Twentieth, Twenty-First and Twenty-Second Annual Reports of the Madison General Hospital*, p. 224. Rules governing interns were amended by the Board of Directors of the Hospital Association, February 16, 1921.

97 *State of Wisconsin Requirements and Recommendations for Accredited Schools of Nursing and for Registration of Nurses* (Madison: State Board of Nursing, 1952), p. 3.

98 *Fourteenth Annual Report of the Madison General Hospital and Training School for Nurses* (1914), p. 11.

99 Minutes of the Sixth Annual Convention of the Wisconsin Hospital Association, November, 1925, Archives, Wisconsin Hospital Association, Madison, Wis.

100 W. H. Smith, "Adequate Medical Service for a Community," *Journal of the American Medical Association* 76 (1921): 1057.

101 Ronald L. Numbers, "The Third Party: Health Insurance in America," in Leavitt and Numbers, eds., *Sickness and Health in America*, p. 142.

102 *Forty-Second Annual Report of the Madison General Hospital* (1942), p. 17a.

103 *Thirty-First Annual Report of the Madison General Hospital and School of Nursing* (1931), p. 26; *Thirty-Fourth Annual Report of the Madison General Hospital and School of Nursing* (1934), pp. 8–9.

104 Numbers, "The Third Party," p. 142.

105 Frank Sinclair, *Blue Cross in Wisconsin* (Racine, Wis.: Western Printing and Lithographing Co., 1965), pp. 23–24; Minutes of the Annual Meeting of the Wisconsin Hospital Association, February 14, 1952, Archives, Wisconsin Hospital Association, Madison, Wis.

106 *Forty-Second Annual Report of the Madison General Hospital*, p. 9.

107 Numbers, "The Third Party," p. 147.

108 *Prospectus, City of Madison, Wisconsin, Hospital Mortgage Revenue Bonds, Series 1969* (Madison, 1969), p. 10.

109 In Wisconsin, except for laws involving contagious and maternity care, hospitals remained fairly autonomous until 1946. The passage of the Hospital Survey and Construction Act (the Hill-Burton Program) and later Medicare and Medicaid, brought increasing federal and state regulation.

110 For a comprehensive discussion of the redistribution of medical personnel, see David L. Brown, "The Redistribution of Physicians and Dentists in Incorporated Places of the Upper Midwest, 1950–1970," *Rural Sociology* 39 (1974): 215–23.

6 *Dale E. Treleven*

One Hundred Years of Health
and Healing in Rural Wisconsin

One day in 1864 a strapping twenty-six-year-old Cornishman descended wearily from a train coach at Fond du Lac. His spirits lifted at the sight of several aunts and uncles, who themselves had immigrated to east central Wisconsin more than two decades before. The railway passenger, my great-grandfather, was among a new wave of Europeans emigrating to the Midwest as the Civil War drew to a close. The Cornishman, not unlike many of the other new settlers, married within the year and began to farm.[1] By 1870 he was harvesting bountiful crops of wheat, oats, and hay to feed his growing family, to provide for the horses, cattle, sheep, swine, and chickens, and to sell in the nearby village of Omro.[2]

Many other settlers also found prosperity and encouraged relatives and friends to join them in the fertile Midwest. But even as thousands of prospective farmers entered Wisconsin and pushed the line of settlement northward, the technological innovations and scientific discoveries that helped bring prosperity to many unleashed other forces that drove even larger numbers from the land and into the cities. Although the absolute number of rural inhabitants in Wisconsin increased annually during the early years of statehood, country dwellers had already begun to decline as a proportion of the state's total population. In 1850, federal census takers found 91 percent of Wisconsin residents living in rural areas. By the eve of the Civil War the percentage stood at about 85, and by 1890 the proportion of Wisconsin inhabitants living in the countryside had fallen to just under two-thirds.[3] Thousands of men and women, boys and girls sought jobs in the very cities and villages that they, or their fathers and mothers, had earlier spurned in favor of a tranquil if challenging hinterland.[4]

At some point between the federal census enumerations of 1920 and 1930, for the first time in the state's history a majority of its residents no longer lived in the countryside.[5] After negligible rural-to-urban migration during the decade of the Great Depression, the impact of technology that followed the Second World War again hastened the movement of farmers and other rural inhabitants to the cities.[6] By 1970 about a third of the state's nearly 4.5 million people remained in rural areas. Although the 20 million acres under cultivation in 1970 equaled the amount of land in farms at the turn of the century, some 65,000 individual farm units disappeared in the same seventy-year period.[7]

The long-term trend of migration to the cities provides a useful context in which to present some observations and make some generalizations about the history of health and healing over the last hundred years in rural Wisconsin. Rural as well as urban inhabitants benefited from the new preventive and curative strategies emerging from scientific investigation and discovery. The development of scientific medicine, particularly during the late nineteenth and early twentieth centuries, led to successful challenges of most of the traditional and often fatal or crippling diseases and illnesses. Although it is difficult to compare a century of medical history in urban and rural areas, it seems clear that such nemeses as typhoid fever, scarlet fever, smallpox, and diphtheria were conquered more or less simultaneously in each. Still, as American society became rapidly urbanized, modernized, industrialized, and specialized, a gap appeared and then widened between rural and urban areas in the availability and accessibility of health care services. As the twentieth century wore on, a chief concern of country people became one of retaining adequate medical services instead of fearing the diseases and plagues of an earlier era.

Settlers in the immediate post–Civil War period found little that resembled the healthful paradise they expected after reading the glowing immigration reports.[8] True, the peaceful prairies and gently rolling hills presented a welcome contrast to the dirt and clutter of Milwaukee, the city through which many passed on their way northward. The new arrivals soon enough learned that sickness and disease regularly crossed political boundaries and wrought havoc among those in the hinterland as well as in the cities. Typhoid fever, typhus, diphtheria, and smallpox, along with pneumonia, measles, scarlet fever, mumps, and other diseases appeared with appalling frequency.[9]

Sickness posed a constant threat. Diphtheria, for instance, in 1863 infected many families in the town of Ellington, in Outagamie County, not long after a smallpox epidemic threatened nearby Appleton.[10] In the late 1870s typhoid fever, a recurring problem where unsanitary conditions prevailed, struck seventy-five citizens and brought death to four at Port Washington, in Ozaukee County.[11] A decade later the secretary of the state board of health, armed with a detailed study of the causes of a typhoid outbreak at Waterford, in Racine County, urged citizens in all communities to implement preventive measures,[12] but the disease continued to rampage across the state through the turn of the century. Diphtheria proved to be especially troublesome. In an outbreak in the early 1880s, of an estimated 10,000 persons affected across the state, more than 2,200 died, many of them in rural areas.[13] A physician in the St. Croix County farming community of New Richmond blamed diphtheria for thirty-four cases of illness and eighteen deaths in one year.[14]

Tuberculosis, commonly associated with cities, also took a heavy toll among rural people well into the twentieth century. For instance, investigators in two widely separated and heavily rural counties, Lafayette and Dunn, found that during the twentieth century's first decade the tuberculosis death rate per 10,000 nearly equaled that of the state as a whole.[15] Incidence of the disease in at least several Dunn County townships equaled that reported for Milwaukee.[16]

The prospect of long and terrifying epidemics in a not-so-healthful rural Wisconsin required that country residents spend a good deal of time, energy, and prayer in attempts to prevent illness and, failing in that, to minimize its effects. A home remedy of one kind or another, often passed from mother to daughter for generations, was usually the first resort when a family member "took sick." Friends and neighbors also provided advice, the specific suggestion depending on the symptoms.[17] Rural people who were able to read English found additional recipes in such popular and diverse guides as the botanic *American Dispensatory*, James Cooper's *Indian Doctor's Indian Receipt Book*, Samuel Thomson's *New Guide to Health*, Samuel Hahnemann's *Organon of Homeopathic Medicine*, or, for female problems specifically, Lydia Pinkham's four-page *Guide for Women*.[18]

Rural Wisconsinites also indulged in packaged, self-dosage medicines and herbs. The printing press was never far behind the line of settlement, and eye-catching advertisements offered alluring remedies for virtually any human ailment. Aspiring small-town newspaper editors, especially after the Civil War, were quick to recognize the economic

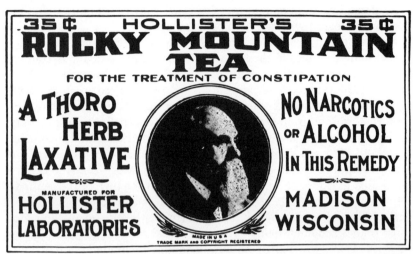

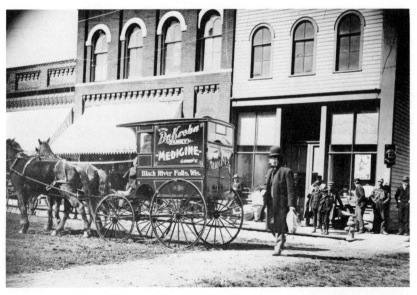

Above: Rural residents often relied on patent medicines, like Hollister's Rocky Mountain Tea, made in Madison. *Below:* Medicine wagons served the small towns and farms of rural Wisconsin.

benefits that patent-medicine advertising brought. Thousands of rural readers learned about the marvelous properties and powers of products with such colorful names as Ayer's Extract of Sarsparilla, Hinkley's Bone Liniment, Hall's Catarrh Cure, and Lydia Pinkham's Vegetable Compound. Religious fundamentalists apparently downed the alcohol-laden concoctions with as much gusto as other users.[19]

When all else failed, a "doctor" was summoned. Rural folks depended on physicians from widely differing backgrounds and with varying degrees of training, skill, and resourcefulness.[20] Regular physicians, sectarian healers, and quacks vied for position.[21] A respected Appleton physician tried to expose his competitors in the press:

Let a man say that he came from some large city, let him rent a house in a respectable street, put on the door in gold letters, "Physician and Surgeon," furnish himself with a case of medicine bottles, buy a horse and buckboard, dress himself invariably in black and drive like Jehu up and down the streets telling everybody who will listen that he has an immense number of patients; let him tell of extraordinary cures he has made, making the slightest cold and sore throat cases of typhoid and diphtheria; let him do all this and you may set it down that he knows nothing about the properties of medicine or the character of disease.[22]

Both poor travel conditions and ageless attitudes towards sickness taxed to the utmost the patience of country doctors in the post-Civil War era. Most rural roads were little more than widened animal paths, rutted and dusty strips that turned into muddy quagmires when it rained.[23] In winter, heavy snowfall and constant drifting complicated the problem of travel. Regardless of season, mode of travel, or the physician's ingenuity, often it took several hours for the doctor to reach his destination after being summoned.[24]

Once he arrived, the country doctor often encountered fear and distrust. The foreign-born, comprising a larger portion of Wisconsin's population than in almost any other state,[25] had habits and customs that often obstructed the good intentions of the physician, frequently native-born and descended from old Yankee stock. A New Richmond doctor in the early 1880s largely blamed the "ignorance and heedlessness of the Irish portion of the residents" for the persistence of an outbreak of diphtheria.[26] The Poles, complained a Trempealeau County physician, were "very hard to manage in sickness," refusing to quarantine themselves when necessary for the good of the community. A physician in Dodge County reported that he tried unsuccessfully to keep the children of the mostly German inhabitants at Hustisford from attending the funeral of a classmate who died of diphtheria; they "resented what they considered my interference," he said.[27]

Not all physicians agreed. A patient, asserted a general practitioner in Bayfield County, knew his insides better than a doctor, and a physician would do well to keep in mind that "a man at forty is a fool or his own physician."[28] But more typical was the complaint of a doctor in Colfax, Chippewa County, who stressed that the Norwegians in his area were next to impossible to treat because they trusted "too extensively to the preacher's rather than to the doctor's directions."[29]

Country doctors had to deal with mental disorder as well as physical illness. As early as the 1860s physicians warned of the effects of the profound desolation and loneliness of the countryside. Dr. W. W. Hall wrote in the first report of the United States Commissioner of Agriculture that the "dairy-maid, so ruddy of cheek, where the roses and the lily vie," was all too often a woman with "pale and wan and haggard face, half covered with long black hair, and coal black eyes peering hotly on you from behind the bars and grates."[30] Wisconsin observers, too, commented on the high incidence of "premature old age and worn out nerves" of farm women. In 1880 a woman speaker informed members of the state agricultural society that premature marriage, motherhood, and overwork commonly added another name to a lengthening "list of farmers' wives who are found in our insane asylums."[31] More often than not the first hospitals in most rural counties housed patients with mental rather than physical illnesses.[32]

Physical illness nevertheless remained the source of the most visible of hardships in the hinterland as well as in the city. Disease, often striking in the form of an epidemic, ultimately brought about a louder general clamor for health reform, especially after the onset of serious economic depression in the 1870s.[33] The Wisconsin legislature voted to establish a state board of health in March 1876, the tenth of its kind in the United States. The Wisconsin board was given broad responsibilities for supervising "the health and life of the citizens of the state" and, more specifically, for setting up a mechanism for health boards in the state's cities and villages to report systematically on illness and death.[34]

While serious sanitation problems in Wisconsin's larger cities had earlier led to the establishment of several local health boards, there had been little organized activity in the hinterland. The popular image of a fragrant Garden of Eden favored with fresh air failed to take into account rural conditions that were all too commonplace: stagnant pools that served as mosquito-breeding grounds, diseased farm animals, unsanitary slaughtering facilities, milk from sick animals, debris-laden house cellars, leaky cesspools, and filthy privy vaults.[35] Members of the state board of health, alarmed at the probable relationship between the unsanitary conditions and sickness, encouraged rural communities to establish health boards to attack the menacing conditions. Some local officials, motivated in part by the board's slogan of "Pure Air, Pure Water, and a Pure Soil," tried to organize community clean-up campaigns.[36] For instance, citizens in the town of Aurora, Waushara County, wanted to drain some of the nearby marshy lands in their diphtheria-ridden neighborhood, but local cranberry growers successfully opposed the idea and a panel of three local doctors decided that the illness came instead from "newly-arrived laborers."[37]

Despite the efforts of the state board of health and a few local health officials who supported community clean-ups, prepared essays such as "The Prevention of Typhoid Fever,"[38] and distributed copies of such pamphlets as "Defence against Cholera and Other Preventable Diseases,"[39] most rural officials would or could do little. A Richland County practitioner, noting that it was impossible to relieve unsanitary conditions because of the "great expense and inconvenience to property owners," reported an increase in typhoid fever at Dayton. Another Richland County physician explained plaintively that his local health board must first "see the fire before they think it needful to call out the engines" of sanitation.[40]

Not all health officials reported bad news. A doctor in Shullsburg, Lafayette County, wrote glowingly of the local board of health, comparing its accomplishments with those of adjoining towns, where "dangerous and contagious diseases are more or less prevalent."[41] More typical, however, was the report of a health official at Elba, Dodge County, which chastised town board members for "thinking that the matter of preventing disease does not amount to much, and being afraid to incur any expense." And while a health officer at nearby Mayville cheered the removal of community slaughterhouses to a location outside the city limits, several hundred miles to the northwest at Hale (Trempealeau County), an official carped about the difficulty of doing much of anything with immigrants who failed to leave in Europe their "old world habits of life."[42]

The failure to curb serious outbreaks of disease led legislators to enact more stringent measures. A serious smallpox epidemic in particular prompted the state legislature to pass a law in 1883 that required each city council and village and town board to appoint a community health board and to select a "reputable physician, whenever possible," as local health officer.[43] The law, which also empowered local officials to report disease to the state as well as the local health board, brought swift action. By 1886 the number of health boards had increased to eleven hundred, a fivefold gain over 1880; by 1895, 1,219 out of 1,256 individual towns, villages, and cities had set up local boards.[44]

The boards performed commendably despite a general lack of citizen support, personnel, and funds. During the late nineteenth and early twentieth centuries, both mortality and morbidity rates declined abruptly in rural areas, as they did in the cities.[45] Scientific medicine brought new preventive and curative measures.[46] Mass programs of inoculation against the traditional nemeses, combined with the enactment and enforcement of stringent sanitary codes and the work of the health boards, all helped to reduce drastically the incidence of various types of disease.[47]

Since the beginning of the twentieth century, the state board of health has published a massive amount of detailed statistics, charts, and graphs documenting the marked decrease in mortality from various types of diseases. Although the data show variations from county to county, the overall decline in the state's rural areas corresponds closely to the rate of decrease in Wisconsin cities. For a sampling of eleven predominantly rural counties, deaths caused by diphtheria declined from 13.1 per 100,000 in 1910 to 1.4 in 1940. During the same period in the same areas, the mortality rate per 100,000 from dysentery, diarrhea, and enteritis fell from 105 to 8, while deaths from typhoid fever dropped from 27 to zero. Deaths per 100,000 attributed to pneumonia declined from 68 to 30 between 1910 and 1940; whooping cough from six to two; and meningitis from 24 to zero.[48]

The data also showed marked reductions in infant and maternal death rates in both rural areas and cities, mainly because public health workers and physicians learned and passed on better information regarding sources of milk and water supplies and nutrition. Statewide infant mortality rates fell by more than 70 percent, from 109 to 29 per 1,000 live births, between 1919 and 1947. During the same period, maternal deaths declined at a similar rate, thanks to better medical care in early stages of pregnancy and growing support from state and national governments for programs to improve obstetrical care.[49]

Rural Wisconsinites began to benefit from the advances in medical science at about the same time other significant improvements took place. New modes of transportation on gradually improving roads, together with a developing telephone system, significantly reduced the isolation of rural people. Communications advances by the second decade of the twentieth century meant, among other things, that country residents could more expeditiously reach a plentiful supply of medical doctors. Wisconsin, according to the national Census Bureau, had 915 physicians and surgeons in 1870, 1,826 in 1890, and 2,684 by 1910. The ratio of physicians and surgeons to population between 1870 and 1910

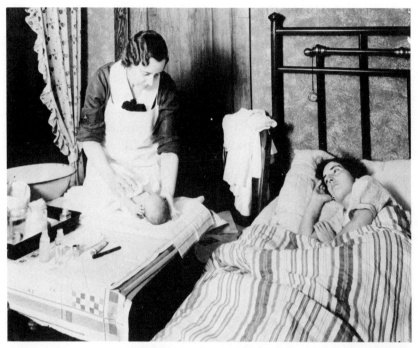

State Historical Society of Wisconsin, WHi(W6)28676

Public health nurses, in an effort to reduce infant mortality, showed urban and rural mothers how to care for their newborn babies.

was very favorable and, as in most other states, the greater proportion of Wisconsin's doctors practiced in rural areas.[50]

After 1910 the physician-to-population ratio grew increasingly unfavorable in rural areas as the focal point of patient care shifted from the bedroom to the hospital. That shift created a new problem for the state's rural people, the effects of which persisted into the 1970s. During the first decades of the twentieth century, urban hospital officials added surgical suites, obstetrics facilities, and diagnostic laboratories, while the hinterland continued to suffer from a shortage of modern buildings and up-to-date equipment. By 1920 there were few hospitals located in Wisconsin's rural areas, except for special-purpose facilities built and subsidized by the state or national government. The federal government, for example, provided hospitals for rural Indians at Hayward, Keshena, Neopit, and Tomah, and the state operated a veterans' hospital in rural Waupaca County. The state of Wisconsin also built hospitals, asylums, and schools for the care of the insane, feeble-minded, and epileptics, mostly in rural areas, while counties also built asylums which were authorized and subsidized by the state legislature.[51]

Despite such facilities, Dr. Charles R. Bardeen, dean of the University of Wisconsin medical school, reported in 1924 that rural Wisconsin had "large areas without [general] hospitals and other areas in which hospital facilities are very limited." This situation persisted partly because the home traditionally had been the site of birth, sickness, and death, and rural citizens felt little inclined to demand modern hospital facilities.[52] Women, for instance, were expected to give birth to their children in the home, attended by a country doctor or by a neighborhood midwife. Indeed, a distinguished academic physician in 1915 reported, after conducting a thorough study of prenatal and natal conditions in Wisconsin, that there was no correlation between infant death and midwife attendance.[53]

As general mortality and morbidity rates declined steadily, in part from mass inoculation efforts, neither state nor local public health authorities needed hospitals to run prevention programs.[54] Nor were hospitals required by the county public health nurses who visited schools to read vital signs and dole out iodine pills for goiter.[55] Moreover, it hardly made sense to locate general hospitals in rural areas at a time when improved transportation provided easier access to urban hospitals.[56] And even if hospitals were close, it was questionable whether the majority of rural sufferers would ignore tradition and permit removal from a sickbed to a hospital.[57]

Of critical importance to rural health, however, was the fact that fewer physicians were willing to practice medicine in communities with inadequate hospital facilities. Medical school graduates, trained in schools whose curricula followed the new standards recommended in the Flexner Report on the status of medical education, felt they should practice in or near cities with proper hospital facilities, up-to-date equipment, and specialized auxiliary personnel. Graduates who, a decade before, were content to practice general medicine, chose to specialize in the 1920s and opted for urban practice.[58]

The First World War affected to some degree physicians' attitudes about the facilities required to practice medicine. More than 750 Wisconsin doctors served in the war, and for the first time many saw the advantages of a nearby hospital or clinic facility.[59] Others witnessed the efficiency of organized ambulance services for transporting sufferers to centralized hospitals far removed from the source of injury. Growing specialization, more exposure to upgraded educational standards, and new first-hand experiences during the war all resulted in fewer medical school graduates who wanted to practice in hinterland communities with inadequate hospital facilities.[60] One physician expressed the nature of the problem with brutal frankness: "The objectionable features of country practice are loss of patients, loss of income, increased expenses, long drives, bad roads, hard work, poorer facilities for practice, no hospitals, no libraries, no laboratories, few churches, poorer schools and loss of time for professional or personal fulfillment."[61]

The research of John Kolb underscored the severity of rural hospital needs by the mid-1920s. Kolb, a young University of Wisconsin sociologist, reported that less than 40 percent of Wisconsin's 114 general hospitals were located in rural communities at a time when over half of the state's people still lived in the open country or in communities of less than 2,500 inhabitants. Only one out of five cities and villages with a population of less than 3,000 had a general hospital; twenty counties, mostly in northern and western Wisconsin, had no general hospital facilities at all.

Kolb also reported that where hospitals did exist in rural communities, more often than not they were poorly equipped. Rural Wisconsin's general hospitals contained only 12 percent of the state's total general hospital beds and fewer still had operating rooms, X-ray machines, or isolation wards. Maternity wards were virtually nonexistent.[62]

Meanwhile, the number of rural physicians declined and the median age of the remaining practitioners steadily increased. From 1910 to 1940 in cities and villages with less than 2,500 people, those with one or more physicians declined from 92 to 71 percent, with the more serious decrease taking place in communities with fewer than five hundred inhabitants. In the same period there was also a decline in rural cities and villages with two or more physicians. In 1910, two-thirds of the rural communities with less than 2,500 inhabitants had two or more doctors; only 40 percent were as fortunate thirty years later. Of the physicians who did remain in rural practice by 1940, a third were at least 60 years of age.[63]

Other studies confirmed that the number of physicians was decreasing in rural Wisconsin. One such survey showed that six overwhelmingly rural counties in western Wisconsin together registered a 20 percent physician loss between 1912 and 1936, although the aggregate population remained the same. During the period, the investigators reported, more doctors moved in than left to practice elsewhere, but those who had died or retired were not replaced. The average age of those who remained in practice within the six-county region increased substantially during the twenty-five-year period, because a large proportion of the most recently graduated medical students located their practices elsewhere.[64]

Undoubtedly, some decrease in service to small villages occurred when physicians moved to other, larger rural communities. Two rural practitioners in Shawano, for example, organized a partnership in 1922, expanded in 1929, and finally constructed a group clinic building three years later.[65] In another case, six physicians in 1916 cooperated to start a group clinic in Marshfield, an important rural Wood County trading center. Rural patients for many miles around had journeyed to the clinic for medical attention by the time the multispecialty group moved into a new building in 1927.[66] Recent medical school graduates and country doctors alike were attracted by the opportunity to begin partnerships or to organize group practices, allowing them ample opportunity to pool their skills and resources in modern, well-equipped ambulatory facilities, located near up-to-date, well-furnished hospitals.

The decline in the number of physicians practicing in rural Wisconsin communities became even more precipitous because of military demands beginning in the early 1940s. Shortly after the Second World War, a rural medical service committee of the American Medical Association joined with an alarmed farmers' group, the Associated Women of the American Farm Bureau Federation, to urge congressional legislation that would help alleviate "the growing scarcity of physicians in farm communities." The committee specifically endorsed legislation to provide funds for the construction and modernization of rural hospitals because "the development in rural communities of centers where diagnostic aids together with public health and other kindred activities could be housed, would attract well trained physicians." Such hospital legislation would not only induce reticent "young physicians to seek locations in the smaller communities," but also improve "the quality of medical practice in rural America without placing the profession in a legislative strait jacket."[67]

In 1946, Congress responded to pressure for better hospital facilities by establishing the Hill-Burton Program. The program required state officials first to set up a hospital survey and construction division within the board of health to assess hospital needs and then to implement a program of construction and modernization.[68] Designers of the Wisconsin Hospital Construction Plan laid out seventy-one hospital areas and assigned to each a priority ranking for funding and construction, after analyzing such factors as the distance of a community from the nearest general hospital as well as various demographic and socioeconomic indicators. State planners assigned a high priority to hospital construction or renovation in rural areas.[69]

By 1952 hospital renovation and construction in rural Wisconsin communities had resulted in a 49 percent increase in the number of hospitals classified by the state board of health as "acceptable" and a 73 percent gain in the number of "acceptable" hospital beds.[70] Residents in and around such rural centers as Boscobel, Osceola, and Lancaster, who had raised the required matching funds, proudly dedicated sparkling new facilities equipped with X-ray units and modern operating, delivery, and patient rooms, all "spotlessly clean and restful."[71] Hospital construction and renovation efforts continued during the rest of the 1950s; by the end of the decade there were only three counties without general hospital facilities.[72]

The gains for rural Wisconsin were significant but modest. Between 1927 and 1960, for instance, the number of general hospitals in communities with fewer than 5,000 inhabitants increased by fourteen, but rural hospitals as a proportion of all the state's hospitals remained about the same. Rural hospital beds as a proportion of all the state's hospital beds increased only slightly in the thirty-three-year period. Planners by 1960 argued that rural communities would need fewer hospitals and beds at a time when nearly 70 percent of Wisconsin's residents, more than a third of whom lived in small towns and open country, remained well outside of metropolitan areas.[73]

From the standpoint of increasing the number of practicing rural physicians, the flurry of hospital modernization activity in the hinterland had little effect. Less than half of the cities and villages with fewer than 2,500 people had one or more physicians in 1960, a marked decrease from 70 percent in 1940. In 1940 two or more physicians practiced in 43 percent of the cities and villages of fewer than 2,500 inhabitants; by 1960 the figure had dropped to 21 percent, with the most drastic decline occurring in the smallest communities. Thus many rural citizens, especially the elderly, found it increasingly difficult to obtain adequate care. The most serious impediments included fewer physicians, increasing population-to-dentist ratios, and the advanced age of many rural physicians.[74]

A national health survey conducted at the end of the 1950s confirmed that the average rural resident received medical assistance less frequently than the city dweller. While the fresh country air no doubt contributed to rural health, rural residents nevertheless were afflicted with as much or more cancer and heart disease as their city cousins. In the case of cancer, while the statewide mortality rate from 1910 to 1960 increased from 66 to 156 per 100,000, the rate for eleven selectively sampled rural counties escalated from 80 to 413 per 100,000 during the same fifty-year span.[75]

Lack of access to, and availability of, adequate medical care services probably led many country people to rely upon the advice and treat-

ments of quacks. Historically, charlatans of one type or another had
found in rural Wisconsin a reliable source of profit. An immigrant log-
ger named John Till, for instance, one day in 1905 emerged from a
woods near Turtle Lake, in Barron County, carrying potent concoctions of plaster salve for open wounds and sores and a mixture of croton
oil and kerosene for all other problems. For a decade thousands of sufferers from one affliction or another sought quick if painful relief at
"Doctor" Till's treatment centers in Barron and St. Croix counties.[76] In
the mid-1950s the operators of an infamous storefront "atomic tunnel"
in Lone Rock (Richland County) proved that rural quackery still thrived
and, indeed, had grown more sophisticated. The uranium "cure,"
though short-lived, drew thousands seeking relief from such maladies as
arthritis and heart disease.[77]

Farm-related medical and health needs remained important in the
modern period. Farming was still the primary economic activity in
much of the Wisconsin hinterland despite the declining proportion of
farm families to the total rural population. Mechanization, a phenome-
non that helped to grow two blades of grass where one had grown before, was also a health scourge.[78] Devices such as the horse-drawn
shredder, with exposed rollers, as early as the turn of the century were
frequently responsible for taking life and limb.[79] Over the years increasingly complex farm machinery became even more hazardous. Large
unwieldy tractors and intricate implements such as corn pickers, balers,
choppers, and combination harvesters (combines) stood out as the most
dangerous. Tractor accidents resulted in nearly 170 deaths from 1960 to
1964, accounting for over 40 percent of the total state farm accident fa-
talities during the period. During the same five-year period, falls
caused another 64 deaths, and farm machinery other than tractors, including power saws, caused 63 deaths.[80] In an all-too-rare but valuable
morbidity study conducted by a rural physician in Trempealeau
County in the mid-1940s, R. L. MacCornack reported that farm-
related incidents caused nearly one-third of all accidents requiring
treatment at his Whitehall clinic.[81]

Animal-borne diseases presented another important hazard in a state
where farmers relied upon dairying or the marketing of animals for well
over half of their gross income.[82] Whatever the merits of the nationwide
vaccination program against "swine flu" during the 1970s, the alarm
over a disease linked to animals served to remind many old-timers of the
last great contemporary epidemic, the influenza epidemic of 1918–1919.
That plague touched even the remotest counties in the state and resulted in an estimated 85,000 cases and more than 11,500 deaths. In
spite of strict preventive measures that prohibited all public gatherings

and closed schools, churches, and theatres, the death rate from influenza and pneumonia, its close companion, at that time reached as high as 500 per 100,000 in many hinterland counties of Wisconsin.[83]

Health-related hazards and problems remained in the 1970s, among them a growing awareness of the possible dangers of herbicides and insecticides,[84] but in general rural Wisconsinites had benefited from modern health care as much as those who lived in the cities. As in the past, patterns of illness in rural and urban environments were characterized more by their similarities than by their differences, except for occupation-related sickness.[85] A continued source of concern and irritation among the state's rural inhabitants was a perceived difference between country and city in the availability and accessibility of medical personnel and facilities. New programs at the state's medical schools, mandated by legislators to educate family physicians who would replace the aging general practitioners in Wisconsin's small cities and villages,[86] brought renewed hope that more, better-trained rural physicians would help to narrow the gap between rural and urban health services.[87] How successful Wisconsin's two specialist-oriented medical schools would be in training a new breed of generalist to meet the needs of those who lived in the Wisconsin hinterland — over a third of the state's population — remained to be seen.

Notes

I am grateful to Clement Imhoff for his outstanding research assistance.

1 *Illustrated Atlas of Winnebago County, Wisconsin*, compiled by George A. Randall (Madison: Brant and Fuller, 1889), p. 31.
2 Manuscript Census of Wisconsin, 1870 (original schedules), 1:340, 2:553–54, State Historical Society of Wisconsin, Madison, Wis.
3 Wisconsin Legislative Reference Bureau, *1975 Blue Book* (Madison: Department of Administration, 1975), p. 695. Definition of rural is that of the U.S. Bureau of Census: open countryside and cities and villages of less than 2,500 population.
4 Walter H. Ebling, *A Century of Wisconsin Agriculture*, Wisconsin Crop and Livestock Reporting Service Bulletin No. 290 (Madison, 1948), pp. 5–6.
5 Walter H. Ebling, *Wisconsin Agriculture in Mid-Century*, Wisconsin Crop and Livestock Reporting Service Bulletin No. 325 (Madison, 1955), p. 3.
6 Walter H. Ebling, *Century of Wisconsin Agriculture*, pp. 4, 17.
7 Wisconsin Statistical Reporting Service, *1975 Wisconsin Agriculture Statistics* (Madison, 1975), p. 6.
8 Wisconsin Board of Immigration, *Statistics: Exhibiting the History, Climate and Productions of the State of Wisconsin* (Madison, 1869), p. 8.
9 Peter T. Harstad, "Disease and Sickness on the Wisconsin Frontier: Smallpox

and Other Diseases," *Wisconsin Magazine of History* 43 (1960): 253–63. Settlers found new frontiers in Wisconsin until after the turn of the century.

10 Lillian Mackesy, "Doctors, Dentists, and Lawyers," in *Land of the Fox: Saga of Outagamie County*, ed. Gordon A. Bubolz (Appleton, Wis.: Outagamie County State Centennial Committee, 1949), pp. 211–12.

11 Wisconsin State Board of Health, *Fourth Annual Report, 1879* (Madison, 1880), pp. 128–33.

12 Wisconsin State Board of Health, *Tenth Annual Report, 1886* (Madison, 1887), pp. 95–107.

13 Cornelius A. Harper, "A History of the Wisconsin State Board of Health," p. 805, manuscript, Archives Division, State Historical Society of Wisconsin, Madison, Wis. Wisconsin State Board of Health, *Eighth Annual Report*, (Madison, 1885), pp. 110–40, is an especially good source on the continuing outbreaks of diphtheria, typhoid, and smallpox for the period from November 1, 1882, to September 30, 1884.

14 Wisconsin State Board of Health, *Seventh Annual Report, 1882* (Madison, 1883), p. 227.

15 Kathrene Gedney, "The Plague on the Farm," *The Crusader*, No. 11 (February 1911), p. 7; Susanne Orton and Jean M. Cook, "A Ten Years' Survey of Tuberculosis in La Fayette County," *The Crusader*, No. 29 (October 1912), pp. 22–26.

16 Hoyt E. Dearholt, "The Survey of Dunn County," *The Crusader*, No. 23 (February 1912), pp. 15–21.

17 Madge E. Pickard and R. Carlyle Buley, *The Midwest Pioneer: His Ills, Cures & Doctors* (Crawfordsville, Ind.: R. E. Banta, 1945), pp. 35–97.

18 Stewart H. Holbrook, *The Golden Age of Quackery* (New York: Macmillan, 1959), pp. 58–66; Adelaide Hechtlinger, comp., *The Great Patent Medicine Era; or, Without Benefit of Doctor* (New York: Grosset and Dunlap, 1970), passim; William Rothstein, *American Physicians in the Nineteenth Century: From Sects to Science* (Baltimore: Johns Hopkins University Press, 1972), pp. 131–40, 152–58.

19 Richard H. Shryock, *Medicine and Society in America, 1660–1860* (New York: New York University Press, 1960), p. 143; Holbrook, *Golden Age of Quackery*, pp. 45–51, 58–66, 157–64. See also James Harvey Young, *American Self-Dosage Medicines: An Historical Perspective* (Lawrence, Kan.: Coronado Press, 1974).

20 Pickard and Buley, *Midwest Pioneer*, pp. 98–166; Rothstein, *American Physicians*, pp. 181–97, 249–81.

21 Shryock, *Medicine and Society*, pp. 150–51. Shryock points out the lack of distinction between well-educated and other practitioners; all were called "doctor."

22 Mackesy, "Doctors, Dentists, and Lawyers," pp. 211–12. On competition between the regular physicians, homeopaths, and eclectics before the turn of the century, see John M. Dodd, *Autobiography of a Surgeon* (New York: W. Neale, 1928), pp. 75–76.

23 William O. Hotchkiss, *Rural Highways of Wisconsin*, Wisconsin Geological and Natural History Survey, Economic Series No. 11, Bulletin No. 18 (Madison, 1906), pp. 77–89.

24 J. V. Stevens, "The Pioneer Wisconsin Family Physician," *Wisconsin Magazine of History* 17 (1934): 337–92; F. G. Johnson, "Experiences of a Pioneer Physician in Northern Wisconsin," *Wisconsin Medical Journal* 38 (1939): 687.

25 *Ninth Census of the United States, 1870* (Washington: Government Printing Office, 1872), 1:ix–xii.

26 Wisconsin State Board of Health, *Seventh Annual Report, 1882*, p. 227.

27 Wisconsin State Board of Health, *Twelfth Annual Report, 1888* (Madison, 1889), pp. 243, 290.

28 Fred G. Johnson, "The Role of the General Practitioner," *Wisconsin Medical Journal* 35 (1936): 391.

29 Wisconsin State Board of Health, *Seventh Annual Report, 1882*, p. 201.

30 W. W. Hall, "Health of Farmers' Families," in *Report of the Commissioner of Agriculture for the Year 1862* (Washington, 1863), p. 462.

31 Helen M. B. Huntley, "Farm Life—Its Hardship and Pleasures," *Transactions of the Wisconsin State Agricultural Society* 19 (1880–81): 255.

32 Bernett O. Odegard and George M. Keith, *A History of the State Board of Control of Wisconsin and the State Institutions, 1849–1939* (Madison: The Board [1940]), passim. For a fascinating if controversial account which touches on mental health in late-nineteenth-century rural Wisconsin, see Michael Lesy, *Wisconsin Death Trip* (New York: Pantheon Books, 1973).

33 Sam B. Warner, Jr., "Public Health Reform and the Depression of 1873–1878," *Bulletin of the History of Medicine* 29 (1955): 503–16.

34 *Laws of Wisconsin, 1876*, Chapter 366; C. A. Harper, "A Brief Outline of Public Health Development in Wisconsin," *Wisconsin Medical Journal* 30 (1931): 803–6.

35 Warner, "Public Health Reform," p. 504.

36 Wisconsin State Board of Health, *Third Annual Report, 1878* (Madison, 1879), p. 38.

37 Wisconsin State Board of Health, *Seventh Annual Report, 1882*, pp. 122–37.

38 Solon Marks, "The Prevention of Typhoid Fever," *Third Annual Report of the Board of Health of the State of Wisconsin, 1878*, pp. 22–29.

39 J. T. Reeve, "Defence against Cholera and Other Preventable Diseases," in Wisconsin Board of Health, *Pamphlets* (Madison, 1885), p. 4.

40 Wisconsin State Board of Health, *Eleventh Annual Report, 1887* (Madison, 1888), pp. 201–2.

41 Ibid., p. 186.

42 Wisconsin State Board of Health, *Ninth Annual Report, 1885* (Madison, 1886), pp. 130–31, 255.

43 *Laws of Wisconsin, 1883*, Chapter 167; Harper, "History of the Wisconsin State Board of Health," p. 52; Wisconsin State Board of Health, *Eighth Annual Report, 1885*, pp. 20–52.

44 L. W. Hutchcroft, "Increasing Health and Happiness of People by Means of Preventive Measures Is Aim of Health Boards," *Wisconsin Medical Journal* 22 (1923–24): 525–27.
45 According to C. A. Harper, during the first thirty years the staff of the state board of health consisted of an executive secretary and one assistant; the annual appropriation had increased to $5,500 by 1905, or $2,500 more than the first appropriation in 1876. See Harper, "A Brief Outline," p. 804.
46 Rothstein, *American Physicians*, pp. 261–81.
47 "Who Killed Cock Robin?" *American Journal of Public Health and the Nation's Health* 34 (1944): 658–59.
48 My sampling of rural counties includes Ashland, Dodge, Forest, Lafayette, Manitowoc, Richland, St. Croix, Shawano, Taylor, Trempealeau, and Waushara; data calculated from annual reports of the Wisconsin State Board of Health from 1910 to 1940. Statewide mortality trends for the same period are conveniently summarized in Wisconsin State Board of Health, *Mortality Statistics, Showing Trend of Certain Diseases of Wisconsin* (Madison, 1942).
49 Wisconsin State Board of Health, *Mortality Statistics, Showing Trend of Certain Diseases of Wisconsin* (Madison, 1944); copy in library of the State Historical Society of Wisconsin includes handwritten data for 1947.
50 *Ninth Census of the United States, 1870*, Vol. 3, *The Statistics of Wealth and Industry of the United States* (Washington: Government Printing Office, 1872), pp. 814–15; *Special Census Report on the Occupations of the Population of the United States, 1910*, Vol. 4, *Population: Occupation Statistics* (Washington: Government Printing Office, 1914), p. 532. There is no reason to believe that Wisconsin was different from many other states in having a much lower proportion of physicians in rural areas in 1960 than it did seventy-five years earlier, an observation made by Shryock, *Medicine and Society*, p. 147, for the country as a whole.
51 Charles R. Bardeen, "Hospitals in Wisconsin," Wisconsin Legislative Reference Bureau, *1925 Blue Book* (Madison: State of Wisconsin, 1925), pp. 235–42. By the mid-1920s Wisconsin's 7,000 beds in thirty-five largely rural counties made it, according to Bardeen, "the leading state in effective care of the chronic insane."
52 Ibid., p. 237.
53 Dorothy R. Mendenhall, "Prenatal and Natal Conditions in Wisconsin," *Wisconsin Medical Journal* 15 (1916–17): 353–69. At the same time, added Dr. Mendenhall, infant mortality rates tended to be higher in the state's rural areas than in the cities.
54 Cornelius A. Harper, "The Work of the State Board of Health, 1876–1924," in Milo M. Quaife, *Wisconsin: Its History and Its People, 1634–1924*, 4 vols. (Chicago: S. J. Clarke, 1924), 2:351–52.
55 Johnson, "Role of the General Practitioner," pp. 393–94.
56 State Highway Commission of Wisconsin and the Public Roads Administration, Federal Works Agency, *Wisconsin Highway Development* (Madison, 1947), pp. 58–59.

57 On the problem of resistance to being moved, see "Wisconsin Physicians Discuss the Problems of the Country Doctor in Several Sections of State," *Wisconsin Medical Journal* 22 (1923–24): 445–46 ff.

58 Ibid.; P. E. Riley, "Are Younger Doctors Going into Country Practice in Wisconsin?" *Wisconsin Medical Journal* 22 (1923–24): 496–97. For the new standards, see Abraham Flexner, *Medical Education in the United States and Canada* (New York: Carnegie Foundation for the Advancement of Teaching, 1910).

59 Fred L. Holmes, "Physicians and Nurses," *Wisconsin Medical Journal* 41 (1942): 134–36. According to Holmes, as of December 1918, 754 of 2,814, or 27 percent, of Wisconsin's physicians had served in the war.

60 J. R. Darnall, "Contributions of the World War to the Advancement of Medicine," *Journal of the American Medical Association* 115 (1940): 1443–51.

61 N. P. Colwell, "Is the Decline of the Country Doctor to Continue? If Not, Why Not, If So, Who or What, Will Take His Place?" *Wisconsin Medical Journal* 22 (1923–24): 325–26 ff.

62 John H. Kolb, "Service Institutions for Town and Country," University of Wisconsin Agricultural Experiment Station, *Research Bulletin*, No. 66 (December 1925), pp. 43–46. A key compilation of contemporary Wisconsin hospital data is "Council on Medical Education and Hospitals of A.M.A. Surveys Wisconsin Hospital Facilities," *Wisconsin Medical Journal* 27 (1928): 242–50, reprinted from data appearing in "Hospital Service in the United States," *Journal of the American Medical Association* 90 (1928): 911–85.

63 Gordon L. Bultena, "The Changing Distribution and Adequacy of Medical, Dental, and Hospital Services in Rural and Urban Communities in Wisconsin, 1910–1960" (Madison: University of Wisconsin, Department of Rural Sociology, 1966), pp. 10, 25.

64 Harold Maslow, "The Characteristics and Mobility of Rural Physicians: A Study of Six Wisconsin Counties," *Rural Sociology* 3 (1938): 267–78.

65 Roger C. Cantwell, "Outline of the Medical History of the City of Shawano, 1850–1956," manuscript, Archives Division, State Historical Society of Wisconsin, Madison, Wis.

66 Marshfield *News Herald*, April 27, 1966.

67 "Report of Committee on Rural Medical Service," *Journal of the American Medical Association* 129 (1945): 1187. In 1946, representatives of farmers' organizations, physicians, dentists, nurses, and state board of health officials in Wisconsin also established a committee to study rural health services. See "Rural Health Education Committee Created at Statewide Conference," *Wisconsin Medical Journal* 45 (1946): 5.

68 U.S. Public Law 79–725, Title VI of the Public Health Service Act, 1946.

69 Wisconsin State Board of Health, "Wisconsin Hospital Construction Plan," mimeographed, with cover letter from Vincent O. Otis, Director, Hospital Survey and Construction Division, November 15, 1947; Charles F. Dahl, "The Federal Hospital Construction Act: A Case Study in Administration"

(M.A. thesis, University of Wisconsin, 1949), pp. 1–2, 15–16, 18, 25–26.

70 Vincent F. Otis, "Does Rural Wisconsin Need More Hospitals?" *Wisconsin Medical Journal* 53 (1954): 334–36 ff.

71 L. O. Simenstad, "The Personal Touch," *Wisconsin Medical Journal* 55 (1956): 1224.

72 Bultena, "Changing Distribution," p. 18.

73 Calculated from *Hospitals* 34, pt. 2 (August 1, 1960), pp. 220–26, and from "Wisconsin Hospital Facilities," *Wisconsin Medical Journal* 27 (1928): 242–50; Wisconsin Legislative Reference Bureau, *1964 Blue Book* (Madison: State of Wisconsin, 1964), p. 84. See C. Horace Hamilton, *Hospitals and Hospital Services in Wisconsin* (Madison: University of Wisconsin, Department of Rural Sociology, 1960), especially pp. 3–8, for a summary of the Wisconsin hospital situation in the late 1950s.

74 Bultena, "Changing Distribution," p. 28. For more information on dentists, see William Stewart, "The Effects of Urbanization on the Distribution of Dental Manpower in Wisconsin," *Journal of the Wisconsin Dental Society* 37 (1961): 121–28.

75 Bultena, "Changing Distribution," p. 26, citing U.S. National Health Survey, *Selected Health Characteristics by Area, Geographic Regions, and Urban-Rural Residence*, July 1957–June 1959, Public Health Service Publication No. 584–C5 (Washington, 1961), pp. 21–25. Data calculations made from *Report of the State Board of Health of Wisconsin, 1910* (Madison, 1911), and Wisconsin State Board of Health, *Wisconsin Public Health Statistics, 1960* (Madison, n.d.), p. 16.

76 Holbrook, *Golden Age of Quackery*, pp. 219–30.

77 Elizabeth Bardwell, "Atomic Quackery: Wisconsin's Uranium Boom," *Wisconsin Magazine of History* 41 (1957–58): 124–31.

78 Ebling, *Century of Wisconsin Agriculture*, p. 82.

79 G. N. Knapp, "Accidents by Farm Machinery," *Twenty-Second Annual Report of the University of Wisconsin Agricultural Experiment Station* (Madison, 1905), pp. 367–73.

80 Wisconsin State Board of Health, *Fatal Farm Accidents, Wisconsin, 1960–1964* (Madison, n.d.), p. 7.

81 R. L. MacCornack, "Rural Accidents," *Wisconsin Medical Journal* 46 (1947): 1118–19. MacCornack found that farm machinery was involved in 20 percent of the total accidents and that "farm work in general" was responsible for another 9 percent. Animal-inflicted injuries — such as dog bites or attacks or kicks from bulls, hogs, or cows — were few. For a summary of farm accident victims who sought care at the Mayo Clinic between 1935 and 1943, see H. Herman Young and Ralph K. Ghormley, "Accidents on the Farm," *Journal of the American Medical Association* 132 (1946): 768–71.

82 Ebling, *Century of Wisconsin Agriculture*, p. 106.

83 Wisconsin State Centennial Committee, *Wisconsin Centennial Story of Disasters and Other Unfortunate Events* ([Madison]: The Committee, 1948), pp. 10–11. Calculations made from the 1918 and 1920 annual reports of the Wisconsin State Board of Health.

84 Thomas R. Dunlap, "DDT on Trial: The Wisconsin Hearing, 1968–1969," *Wisconsin Magazine of History* 62 (1978): 3–4.
85 Frederick D. Mott and Milton I. Roemer, *Rural Health and Medical Care* (New York: McGraw-Hill, 1948), pp. 87–113.
86 *Wisconsin Assembly Bulletin, Regular Session, 1969*, pp. 612–13 (Assembly Bill 1172).
87 American Medical Association, Ad Hoc Committee on Education for Family Practice, *Meeting the Challenge of Family Practice* ([Chicago], 1966), passim. The most complete status report on Wisconsin's general practitioners/family physicians as of 1970 is John H. Renner, Dale E. Treleven, and Virginia F. Lienhard, "An Inventory of Family Physicians in the State of Wisconsin: Practice Arrangement, Age, and Distribution" ([Madison]: University of Wisconsin Family Practice Program, 1972).

7 Judith Walzer Leavitt

Health in Urban Wisconsin:
From Bad to Better

It has been said that Wisconsin has only one city—Milwaukee. Throughout the state's history the metropolis on Lake Michigan has far outranked other urban centers in Wisconsin in size and diversity of population, in economic strength and complexity, and in cultural amenities. Consequently, it has come to epitomize urban life in Wisconsin and therefore logically serves as the focus of this chapter.

Nevertheless, we should bear in mind that Wisconsin's other urban centers—Madison, Racine, Green Bay, Kenosha, Oshkosh, Superior, La Crosse, Sheboygan, and Fond du Lac—were often as important to their respective regions as Milwaukee was to the state as a whole. Their relatively dense populations, industrial and commercial economies, and urban life-styles set them apart from their rural surroundings. In 1891 a resident of Fond du Lac described life in his "city" of 15,000: "The busy bustle of its crowded ways, bordered with thriving stores or charming residences, the mills, factories and foundries that make incessant stir, the ceaseless industry that makes the freight houses and depots continually seethe like enormous hives in swarming time, all speak convincingly of enterprise and prosperity."[1] Clearly, persons living in such environments had more in common with the citizens of Milwaukee than with neighboring farmers.

Like other American cities in the mid-nineteenth century, Wisconsin's cities faced a multitude of health problems. While general mortality rates in the United States remained fairly stable, urban rates were increasing.[2] Conditions of urban life seemed to exacerbate health problems. Infectious diseases that seldom reached isolated regions spread rapidly through crowded urban areas. Commercial cities invited new diseases with each boat or train arriving from other parts of the nation and provided ideal conditions for their multiplication. Crowded, dark, unventilated housing, unpaved streets mired in horse manure and littered with refuse, inadequate or nonexistent water supplies, privy vaults that remained unemptied from one year to the next, stagnant pools of water, ill-functioning open sewers, and an overwhelming stench characterized America's cities. The population explosion and large-scale industrialization of the late nineteenth century greatly accentuated these negative aspects of the urban environment, which threatened life and health.

Of all Wisconsin cities, Milwaukee held the greatest health dangers for the urban dweller. Rapid population growth in the last part of the nineteenth century overwhelmed the city, which was unprepared for the influx. New immigrant families crowded into single rooms or basement hovels. Tenement conditions in Milwaukee never matched those in New York City for density and squalor, but in the frame cottages on the southwest side, and in similar pockets throughout the city, lived far too many people with too few sanitary facilities.[3]

Contemporary Milwaukee observers noted the effects of overcrowding and basement living on people's health. Medical practitioners felt overwhelmed in their attempts to stem the tide of disaster when epidemics spread through densely populated wards. Not only was isolation impossible, but adequate ventilation, cleanliness, and proper diet remained beyond the reach of most families. As late as 1893 one physician discussed the futility of treating diphtheria in the poorer sections of the city: "We might as well confess it right straight off, that we just have to give up. We have to give up because of the local surroundings over and over again."[4]

High death rates among children indicated the extent of the problem. A health officer in Milwaukee lamented the fact that children under five years of age (who formed approximately 12 percent of the total population) accounted for 61 percent of the deaths in the city. "This slaughter of innocents," he noted in 1872, "is found, chiefly, in crowded parts of the city, where families are massed together, in filthy, dark, ill-ventilated tenements, surrounded by dirty yards and alleys, foul privies, and imperfect drainage. In such an atmosphere, the child inhales a deadly miasmatic poison in every breath it draws."[5] A statistical

study of Milwaukee's tenements in 1905 showed that intractable housing problems persisted into the twentieth century: Milwaukee's poorest
lived in back-to-back tenements plagued by inadequate ventilation,
faulty drainage, and sewage back-ups, or crowded into wet and reeking
basements.[6]

Housing was a major problem, but other aspects of the urban environment also helped create the city's poor health record. A stroll down a
Milwaukee street offended eyes, nose, and ears. Urbanites encountered
horse manure in large quantities everywhere. According to one estimate
from the 1890s, a single horse dropped about 15 pounds of manure on
urban streets every 24 hours.[7] On a rainy day the manure mixed with
mud and trash from the unpaved or littered streets, and pedestrians un-
avoidably picked it up on shoes and clothing. Dead horses lay for days,
if not weeks, where they had fallen. Garbage was frequently left out or
dumped in the streets, where scavenger pigs consumed it or "swill children" collected it.[8] One observer in the 1880s noticed that garbage remained so long on Milwaukee streets that it had the "audacity to attempt to remove itself, by crawling away, in the shape of active little
worms, to the great consternation and disgust of all housewives . . .
and to the detriment of the general health of the city."[9] Urban smells
compounded the problem. One Milwaukeean wrote of his evening walk
in 1866: "Last evening a gentle southwest breeze was blowing across the
city, and wafted the most delicious odors imaginable from the *slaughter
houses*. . . . Decayed animal matter commingled with the aroma from
the marsh, forming a perfume which for *strength* if not for *sweetness*
could not be excelled even in Chicago, the famed city of smells."[10] Full
privy vaults further enhanced the urban stench and permeated the
ground to contaminate the water supply from nearby wells. Unflushed
open sewers added to the odor and unsightliness of urban streets. Milwaukee streets were frequently impassable because of the accumulation
of refuse, garbage, manure, and dead animals.

Such environments spawned many diseases and kept death rates
high. Milwaukee's biggest killer in the nineteenth century was tuberculosis, which accounted for more deaths in the city than any other single
disease.[11] The urban environment proved particularly conducive to the
spread of tuberculosis. Crowding, shared drinking and eating utensils,
and unsanitary facilities fostered its spread. Typically, tuberculosis
caused 10 to 14 percent of Milwaukee deaths. Diarrheal diseases (cholera infantum, "summer complaint," and dysentery) represented the second highest cause of death in the city, responsible for 8 to 10 percent of
mortality. These diseases spread through excreta under conditions of inadequate sanitary facilities, or through water or milk contamination.

Another major cause of death was the dreaded diphtheria. With fatality rates as high as 44 percent of cases, and with symptoms of alarming character, this disease ranked among the most feared scourges of childhood. It spread, through oral and nasal secretions, particularly rapidly under crowded urban conditions. Other diseases that the urban environment cultivated included pneumonia, scarlet fever, and typhoid fever.

The distribution of Milwaukee's mortality among the various wards and sections of the city offers an indication of which groups were most severely affected by illness. The most populous immigrant wards suffered the highest mortality rates. The wards in which significant numbers of native-born Americans lived remained below the mean for death rates. In 1898, for example, infant mortality, diarrheal diseases, and tubercular diseases were all more prevalent in the immigrant wards (Poles in the South Side and Germans in the North Side) than anywhere else. The wards that had the highest resident density consistently sustained the highest mortality in the city in the nineteenth and the early twentieth centuries.[12] The highest mortality rates repeatedly occurred in the South Side's fourteenth and eleventh wards, where large numbers of Polish immigrants lived. Crowded into small homes, these victims of poverty could not afford to install sewer or water pipes that might have aided their plight. High mortality in the North Side German wards, less congested and less impoverished than the Polish wards, can be explained in part by cultural patterns of resistance to vaccination and other public health measures that involved governmental control over personal lives.[13]

Congestion within urban dwellings (measured by number of people per house) correlated closely with mortality from infectious diseases in Milwaukee. In 1890 and in 1900 a high positive correlation can be shown between the variables of housing density and general mortality. As the number of persons within a Milwaukee dwelling increased, mortality increased.[14]

Health statistics reveal that while mortality was greatest in areas of high population density, incidence of disease encompassed the city: all Milwaukee wards, rich and poor, native and immigrant, had problems with infectious diseases. Clearly attributable to the urban environment as well as to the state of medical knowledge and availability and use of medical facilities, the spread indicates that no one was safe from urban diseases or free from the anxiety of premature death.

Milwaukee was not the only city in Wisconsin to suffer from dangerous environmental conditions and high mortality rates. All of its urban centers complained of conditions conducive to the spread of disease in the nineteenth and early twentieth centuries. A Green Bay correspondent to the state board of health, in trying to explain that city's high mortality rates in 1881, wrote that "the general drainage . . . is so poor that it is a matter of surprise that we are not more severely scourged [by disease than we are]."[15] He attributed whatever health Green Bay enjoyed to the salubrious lake breezes that counteracted the urban influence.

Sheboygan residents, too, identified the poor sanitary condition of their streets and homes as a constant source of danger to health. "Sheboygan is growing rapidly and everything in the shape of a house, no matter what its sanitary condition may be, is occupied often to overcrowding, in the case of the poorer classes." The city's health officer, overwhelmed by the extent of the problem, queried helplessly, "What can be done?"[16]

Madison's board of health made over one thousand investigations into filthy conditions in the city during 1885. Its health officer, with suitable understatement, reported that "the city in general did not offer a particularly cleanly appearance."[17] Observers in all cities noticed that conditions were particularly offensive in the most crowded poorer parts of town, where the negative aspects of urban life were concentrated.

Rural residents contrasted the unhealthy condition of Wisconsin's cities with the seemingly healthy isolation and clean air of the country. The health official in Naples filed the following report in 1885: "The population being entirely farmers, we have been remarkably free from diphtheria, typhoid fever and similar diseases. We have no cases of diarrhea or dysentery and there is no contagious disease in the township."[18] Indeed, someone in Fountain bragged in the same year, "People seldom die of anything except old age here."[19] The apparent contrast with rural Wisconsin merely accentuated the problems urbanites faced in the last half of the nineteenth century. Their homes, their places of work, their very surroundings threatened their lives every day. Escape seemed impossible.

Individual city dwellers could not control the pervasive sanitation problems that plagued their lives. If they kept their property clean, collected their garbage, emptied their privies, and purified their well water, they still remained vulnerable to contamination by others. Especially in the crowded wards of the city, individuals were at the mercy of their neighbors. Unable to control communal behavior, urbanites could only wait for the city government to come to their aid, a process that gradually evolved after the 1870s.

Milwaukee, with the most pressing problems and the greatest resources, led the way. A rapidly expanding population (approximately

71,000 in 1870) forced Milwaukee to recognize the extreme health dangers that prevailed in the city. In 1867 it established a board of health modeled on New York City's metropolitan board and hired a physician to begin the job of making Milwaukee a healthier place in which to live. The Milwaukee Board (later Department) of Health initiated sanitation campaigns, including garbage and dead animal collection and disposal, water supply and sewerage systems, and street sweeping — proudly, if gradually, increasing its control over the urban environment. Although simple cause-and-effect relationships are hard to document, most of the new measures instituted in the name of public health did improve the health potential of urbanites.

Milwaukeeans early recognized the relationship between water supplies and health problems. Citizens obtained water from private wells and cisterns, from the few public wells, or from the rivers that ran through the city. But the growing population and nascent industrialism contaminated the rivers and wells with "effete matter," making them "dangerous to life." The city needed a more bountiful and healthful supply.[20] In 1868 Milwaukee commissioned Ellis Sylvester Chesbrough, the nationally famous engineer who had fashioned Chicago's water and sewerage system, to design a water works. Chesbrough's plan was to draw clean Lake Michigan water into pipes and distribute it throughout the city.[21] A debate about the cost of the project delayed building of the water works until 1874. When the system was finally finished, the Board of Health jubilantly called attention to the benefits of the new and clean source of water: "There is no city in the Union better supplied with pure water than Milwaukee."[22]

Unfortunately, not all Milwaukeeans benefited from this new boon. Citizens had to pay for their connections to the town lines. Many Milwaukeeans, particularly the poorer new arrivals who already suffered heavily from infectious diseases, could not afford to pay for the laying of pipes or the water rates. Despite the inequities, by 1876 64 miles of pipe had been laid and by 1884 over 110 miles of water pipes were buried under Milwaukee's streets.[23]

A second problem developed with Milwaukee's "newest blessing" — one that Chesbrough himself had anticipated but one for which he had not made adequate provision. Because of the proximity of the water intake to the city's sewer outlet in Lake Michigan, Milwaukee's new supply of water soon showed signs of contamination. Quantities of raw sewage entered the lake daily, and city officials occasionally dumped city garbage into the lake as well. The resulting pollution threatened those who drank city water, especially when bad weather churned up the lake waters. Asking "Do we drink our own excreta?" one newspaper

answered that Milwaukeeans drink "a decoction of uncertain propor-
tions of Milwaukee river, Milwaukee sewage, Menomonee Marsh,
slaughterhouses, breweries, and tanneries."[24] Another reporter warned
simply: "There is death in our drink."[25]

In repeated attempts to improve this intolerable situation, the health
commissioner called the "pouring of millions and millions of gallons of
untreated sewage daily into the water upon which the people of this
city depend for drinking" an "unspeakably filthy and crude" habit. He
predicted a "harvest of . . . calamity" unless the situation were reme-
died.[26] Finally confronting the problem, the city began systematically
treating the water with purifying chemicals in 1912. Although positive
results were sometimes slow in coming, municipal efforts such as the
water supply systems helped the lives of urbanites. By working collec-
tively, individuals trapped in the increasingly complex urban morass
gradually shaped their environment to meet their health needs.

Under Chesbrough's plan for the water system, sewage emptied daily
into Milwaukee's three rivers on its way to the lake. The rivers sent up
summer odors, the unhealthfulness of which was widely acclaimed in
the daily press. "The Milwaukee River is getting to be a stench in the nos-
trils of the people," proclaimed one. The health commissioner agreed
that the Menomonee River was "an open sewer of the vilest character."[27]
Another health official described Burnham's Canal, which received the
outpourings of the city's distilleries and slaughterhouses, this way:

The thick, inky, putrid water of the canal could be seen in many places in a state
of violent commotion, produced by the fermentation existing at the bottom. . . .
so noxious was the fermentating matter, that the water, grains, cow manure,
and other filthy matter was thrown by the power and explosive force of gas gen-
erated, many feet into the air. This agitation of the water and evolution of gas
continued over a large surface of the canal, and resembled what might result
from some great subterranean explosive power.[28]

A series of flushing tunnels that kept the channels flowing during the
dry summer months finally controlled the river nuisance. But not until
well into the twentieth century did a more sophisticated system incorporate intercepting sewers to allow the sewage to bypass the rivers entirely and sewage treatment to keep lake pollution at a minimum.

Another related urban sanitation problem concerned privy vaults,
which remained in common use in Milwaukee throughout the nineteenth century. The Health Department found foul privies on virtually
every block in the city, most of them without cement floors or water-
tight walls. Although officials licensed the private scavengers who typically collected the "night soil," they did nothing about instituting public

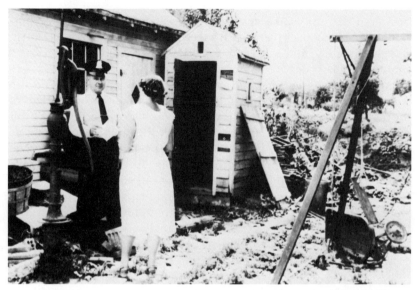

Courtesy of City of Milwaukee Health Department

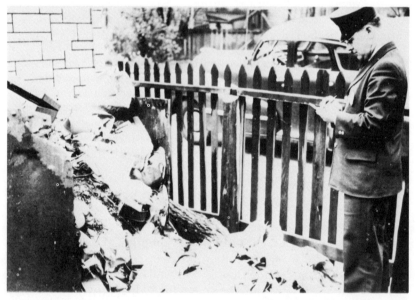

Courtesy of City of Milwaukee Health Department

For years the Milwaukee Health Department hired sanitary inspectors to certify outhouses and to issue citations for uncollected garbage and refuse.

collection of human excrement. "The removal of night soil is essentially a private matter. . . . There is no obligation upon the city to remove night soil," proclaimed one newspaper editorial.[29] Not until water closets replaced privies (beginning in the 1870s but not completed until the mid-twentieth century) did Milwaukee solve the privy nuisance.

Ironically, some of the improvements sought by urban health departments led to new frustrations for individual urbanites. For example, when a city developed water and sewerage systems in its effort to improve sanitation, it introduced the fear of contamination by sewer gas. Decomposition of organic material would, according to this popular nineteenth-century theory, emit an invisible and odorless gas that carried with it a disease-producing potential. Sewer gas in Milwaukee was thought to be "worse than a corpse in a house." One sanitarian noted: "To-day it brings with it the contagion of typhoid; to-morrow it introduces diphtheria; next day it smuggles in scarlatina. It gives no warning, and its unknown presence is not shunned. It sleeps with you, creeps into every cell of your lungs, and lays shadowy fingers on every drop of your heart's blood."[30] Homeowners feared the dangers so much that some felt safer without connection to the public sewers.[31] It is impossible to judge the actual effects that sewer gas might have had on health, but many nineteenth-century physicians firmly believed that the introduction of sewer pipes compounded health problems rather than lessened them.

In a related area of sanitation, garbage, the Milwaukee Health Department became preoccupied with the questions of collection and disposal in the last thirty years of the nineteenth century. The "nightmare" of garbage created more "trouble and annoyance" than any other problem faced by the health officials.[32] Because most physicians believed that dirt caused disease, sanitary garbage disposal became the symbol of the movement to clean up the city and make it more healthful. Until the Health Department involved itself in garbage collection, Milwaukee streets were "perfect avenues of swill" and a "disgrace to the city."[33] Repeatedly newspapers and health officials blamed garbage for the high mortality rates in the city, especially during the summer months. The Health Department began to regularize collection in 1875; by 1880 it spent more of its budget on garbage than on all other health-related activities combined, and the figure kept rising.[34] Despite all the money and time invested, Milwaukee did not easily solve the tremendous problem of collecting and disposing of increasing amounts of solid waste materials. The city experimented with all the known methods of garbage disposal, including using it for pig food, selling it for land fill, dumping it into Lake Michigan, rendering it into fertilizer and grease, and totally cremating it. Not knowing the best alternative and repeatedly voicing their confusions, health officials found themselves at the mercy of politicians who sought to use the garbage jobs — collectors, inspectors, and engineers — as patronage plums. Relentlessly trying new techniques as they became available and fighting local forces unconcerned with the health implications of rotting garbage, the Milwaukee health commissioners finally established a municipal cremation plant in 1902 and "permanently solved the waste disposal problem."[35] This plant and its 1910 replacement served Milwaukee until 1955.

Urbanites also found it difficult to control the quality of their food. At the mercy of the producers and distributors who offered tainted or old food in the marketplace, they had few alternatives to buying it. Meat was one key problem. Animals were slaughtered under appalling conditions, and health officials, reluctant to appear "hostile to any branch of trade" that brought wealth to Milwaukee, had a difficult time controlling this industry, which produced both a local sanitary nuisance and a menace to those who tried to consume the product. One slaughtering house reportedly processed meat near "the head and intestines of an animal . . . lying on the floor for at least one week and within six feet of the remains of a large rat . . . lying lifeless on its back." Until the national campaign to regulate meat-packing in 1906 gave the local officials a boost, there was little they could do about such establishments.[36]

Milk posed similar problems, because it spoiled rapidly, especially during the summer months. In rural areas people were close to the milk supply and could be ensured of a relatively fresh product. But city dwellers did not have easy access to milk in the nineteenth century. Not only did most milk travel long distances to reach consumers, but it often was contaminated by the time it arrived. Milk was one of the most significant hazards of urban childhood. High child mortality rates testified to its dangers.

The urban cow barn offered the worst of conditions. Milwaukee's health commissioner uncovered an appalling situation in the city's stables in 1882. In one he noted:

Pools of noxious water and refuse covered the floor, which was soft and soaked with foul liquid. The eight cows stood closely tied, their sides touching. None were lying down, and it did not look as though they could, without crowding upon each other, although their quarters and flanks, that were thickly coated with manure, showed that they did change their positions. Their hides were damp with sweat, and several were panting laboriously.[37]

City milk drinkers had little choice in milk selection. Unable to see

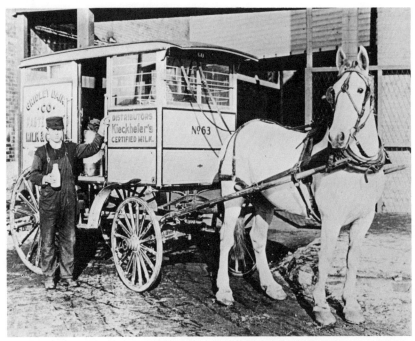

State Historical Society of Wisconsin, WHi(W6)21070

Early in the twentieth century the Gridley Dairy in Milwaukee began distributing certified milk, that is, raw milk from tuberculosis-free cows, bottled under sanitary conditions.

any difference between one product and another, they often chose the cheapest. Health officials worked hard to alleviate unsanitary conditions in cow barns and dairies that endangered the public welfare. Gradually, municipalities in Wisconsin acquired powers to regulate the purity of the milk sold within their boundaries and to make available to the urban consumer a potable and relatively healthful product. During the late nineteenth and the early twentieth centuries local Wisconsin health departments increasingly controlled milk-borne infections. In 1912 in La Crosse, for example, the health officer traced all cases of scarlet fever to one milk route. "We stopped the sale of milk on that route for a week," he reported, "and at the same time the outbreak of scarlet fever stopped and we had no more of it."[38] Rapidly declining infant mortality rates give some evidence that the efforts of health departments were not in vain (see Figure 7.1).[39]

Other attempts to solve urban health problems also met with success at the turn of the twentieth century. Increasing power to control diseases greatly lessened both incidence and mortality from some of the

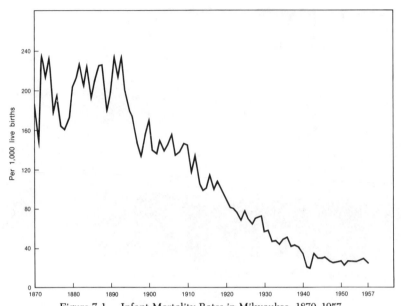

Figure 7.1.   Infant Mortality Rates in Milwaukee, 1870–1957
Source: Milwaukee Health Department Annual Reports, 1870–1908, and Division of Vital
Statistics Records, located in the Milwaukee Health Department Division of Vital Statistics.

most severe contagious diseases, such as smallpox or diphtheria, indicating ways in which health officials could utilize advancing medical
knowledge in the urban setting. In Milwaukee and in most of the other
Wisconsin urban areas, smallpox vaccination and later diphtheria antitoxin were freely available and widely distributed to all who needed
them. Availability, of course, did not guarantee use, and Wisconsin's
cities illustrated the complex interrelationships between medical
knowledge, cultural beliefs, and politics evident elsewhere. A strong
antivaccination group in Milwaukee was successful in limiting the use
of the smallpox preventive until the twentieth century. Likewise, skep-
tics insured a slow acceptance of diphtheria antitoxin after its introduction in 1894. However, the Health Department quickly secured some
New York antitoxin in January 1895 and established free distribution
stations around the city for the sick poor.[40]
    Although city life could be bleak indeed in Victorian America, urban
health began improving by the end of the nineteenth century. Decreasing mortality statistics indicate the trend and illustrate that the gap between urban and rural was closing. (see Figure 7.2). In part the general
improvement indicated by these statistics is a function of the accomplishments of boards of health and improved urban services. The num-

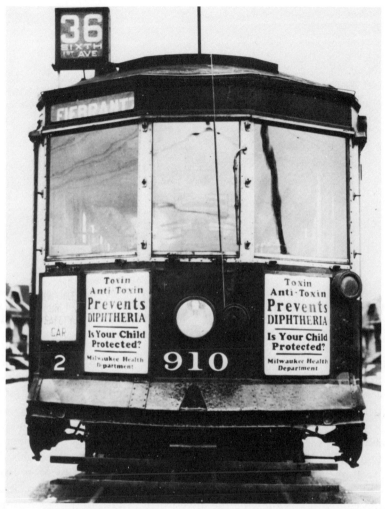

Courtesy of City of Milwaukee Health Department

In 1928 the Milwaukee Health Department mounted posters on city streetcars urging parents to inoculate their children against diphtheria.

ber of local boards and the scope of health department activities increased in the last quarter of the nineteenth century and throughout the twentieth century. La Crosse and Kenosha joined Milwaukee in hiring full-time public health officers who could devote the necessary energy to conquering the problems created in the cities. Because the problems were greatest in large population centers, cities initiated the preventive

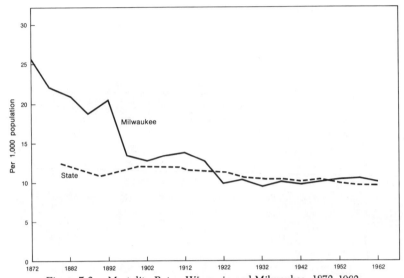

Figure 7.2.   Mortality Rates, Wisconsin and Milwaukee, 1872–1962.
Sources: Milwaukee Health Department, Annual Reports, 1870–1908, and Division of Vital
Statistics Records, located in the Milwaukee Health Department Division of Vital Statistics;
Wisconsin State Board of Health Annual Reports, 1880–1940, and Bulletins, 1950–1962.

measures that helped lead to better health statistics throughout the
state.[41] Among the most important contributions health boards made to
lowering death rates were improved control over the production and
distribution of such foods as milk, meat, and bakery goods; increased
control over sanitation, including water, sewerage, and garbage collection and disposal; regulation of privies and private wells; enforcement
of housing and building codes; and increasingly effective measures of
controlling the spread of infectious diseases. By 1910 Milwaukee had
improved its health record well enough to stand among the seven cities
in the United States showing the lowest death rates. In the second and
third decades of this century, Wisconsin's other cities followed Milwaukee's example and significantly improved their health standards.

As we have already seen, health reforms were not accomplished easily.
Despite the now obvious connection between public health measures
and improved health statistics, these benefits were not always evident
to people at the time. Conflicting interests clashed over what was the
best reform, how to institute it, how to pay for it, and how to distribute
its benefits. No reform, not even providing clean milk for urban babies,
passed without a fight or without groups believing that another solution, or no governmental action at all, would be preferable. The struggle for health reform, which this chapter has briefly surveyed, was

complex and intricate. Physicians frequently disagreed about the importance of a given reform; laypeople found it even more difficult to evaluate the various proposals. The political milieu and conflicting economic interests further complicated the process.[42] Although Wisconsin cities gradually achieved some control over their environments and over the health of their inhabitants, they did not do so with any clear sense that they chose the only right direction or with the full support of their populace. They inched along, groping for possible solutions that often appeared as murky as the putrid matter they attempted to eliminate.

The question remains: Was it healthier for a person to live in the city or in the rural areas? The answer varies considerably over time. In the last third of the nineteenth century, urban health problems were most severe, and solutions were only beginning to be discovered. During that period cities attempted to cope with greatly expanding populations, increasing industrialization, and enormous social and health-related problems that descended rapidly upon them. During that time urban residents were at greater risk for illness and death than their rural counterparts. Higher mortality rates testify to the dangers of urban life. Precisely because urban problems were greater, city dwellers put more effort into finding solutions. In time the efforts of local health departments produced results, both in preventing diseases and in curing them. Some of these were medical and therefore applicable in rural areas as well. Others were specifically urban, developed to combat such problems as sanitary garbage disposal and purification of water systems. Mortality rates of both urban and rural areas responded to advancing measures and show decreases beginning in the late nineteenth century. But urban mortality rates dropped faster than rural mortality rates. By the 1920s mortality statistics indicated that it was as healthy to live in Wisconsin cities as it was to live in its hinterlands (see Figure 7.3).

In terms of access to professional medical care and institutions, living in cities consistently ranked above living in rural areas. At the turn of the twentieth century over 50 percent of the public and private hospitals in the state were located in the state's ten most populous cities, which contained only 20 percent of the population.[43] Not only were there more facilities to use in case of illness, but the public institutions that provided medical care for citizens free of charge (with the exception of tuberculosis sanatoriums and insane asylums) were uniformly located in urban areas. In the 1870s Milwaukee became the first Wisconsin city to build a hospital specifically to provide charity care for the sick poor; other cities followed as their populations increased.

Living in a city also increased one's chances of having access to a physician, opportunities that improved over the course of the twentieth century (see Figure 7.4). The presence of physicians did not insure

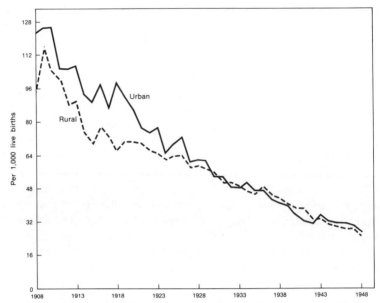

Figure 7.3. Urban and Rural Infant Mortality Rates in Wisconsin, 1908–1948
Source: Wisconsin State Board of Health Annual Reports, 1908–1948.

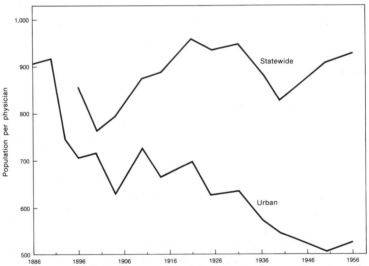

Figure 7.4. Statewide and Urban Ratio of Physicians to Population in Wisconsin,
1886–1956
Sources: *Polk's Medical and Surgical Register of the United States and Canada*, 1886–1914;
*American Medical Directory: A Register of Legally Qualified Physicians in the United
States and Canada*, 1921–1956.

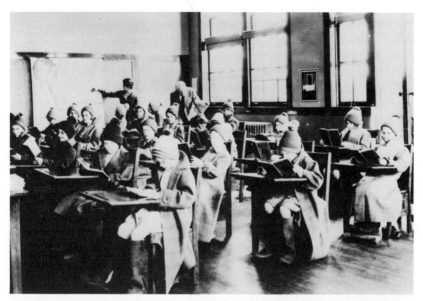

Courtesy of City of Milwaukee Health Department

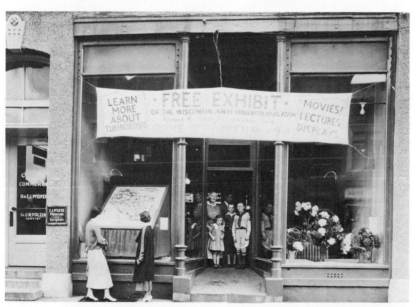

State Historical Society of Wisconsin, WHi(X3)9573

Above: As part of its anti-tuberculosis campaign in the early 1930s, Milwaukee ran a fresh-air school on Oklahoma Avenue. *Below:* During the 1920s the Wisconsin Anti-Tuberculosis Association used Christmas Seal money to send traveling exhibits around the state.

treatment or cure, but public facilities available in urban areas allowed many urbanites to obtain medical aid in the event of sickness.

Wisconsin cities proudly noted in 1926 that their health improvements compared well with cities throughout the country. On the basis of a low incidence of communicable diseases, infant hygiene, school health, sanitation, and laboratory facilities, Kenosha and Oshkosh stood among the top 29 cities nationwide in the American Public Health Association's Better Cities Contest.[44] The APHA repeatedly awarded Milwaukee the title of "healthiest" large city in the nation in the 1930s, and in the 1940s it gave Wisconsin's largest city a place in the National Health Honor Roll.[45] State efforts to improve urban health and hygiene, efforts that were begun under desperate urban conditions in the nineteenth century, paid dividends in the improving statistics of the twentieth century.

Notes

I would like to thank Rima D. Apple and Deanna Reed Springall for their research assistance in the preparation of this paper.

1 *Fond du Lac Illustrated* (Milwaukee: Art Gravure & Etching Co., 1891), p. 6.
2 Frederick L. Hoffman, "American Mortality Progress during the Last Half Century," in *A Half Century of Public Health*, ed. Mazyck P. Ravenel (New York: American Public Health Association, 1921), p. 101.
3 For descriptions of three sample Milwaukee wards, see Roger David Simon, "The Expansion of an Industrial City: Milwaukee, 1880–1910" (Ph.D. diss., University of Wisconsin, Madison, 1971).
4 Dr. A. B. Farnham, during a discussion at a meeting of the Milwaukee Medical Society, April 25, 1893. Minutes of the society are in the Milwaukee Academy of Medicine.
5 M. P. Jewett, president of the Board of Health, in *Fifth Annual Report of the Board of Health of the City of Milwaukee Comprising Remarks on Sanitary Requirements, with Returns of Deaths for the Year Ending April 1, 1872* (Milwaukee: Yewdale Printer, 1872), p. 7. Hereafter Milwaukee Board of Health and Health Department annual reports will be cited MHD, *Annual Report*.
6 "The Housing Problem in Wisconsin," *Twelfth Biennial Report of the Bureau of Labor and Industrial Statistics, State of Wisconsin, 1905–1906* (Madison: Democrat Printing Co., 1906), pp. 275–334.
7 See Joel A. Tarr, "Urban Pollution Many Long Years Ago," *American Heritage* 22 (1971): 65–69 ff.
8 For an interesting short account of Milwaukee's swill children, see Charles D. Goff, "The Swill Children of Milwaukee," *Historical Messenger* (Milwaukee County Historical Society), March 1960, pp. 9–11.

9 *Proceedings of the Common Council of the City of Milwaukee for the Year Ending April 16th, 1889* (Milwaukee: Ed. Keogh, 1889), July 16, 1888, p. 168.

10 Milwaukee *Sentinel*, October 17, 1866, p. 1.

11 This and subsequent discussion of the diseases that attacked Milwaukee are based on Judith Walzer Leavitt, "Public Health in Milwaukee, 1867–1910" (Ph.D. diss., University of Chicago, 1975). See particularly Table 2: Milwaukee Mortality Statistics, pp. 24–27, derived from the Milwaukee Health Department's annual reports and its Bureau of Vital Statistics.

12 See ibid., pp. 30–43; and Simon, "Expansion of an Industrial City," p. 227.

13 More study needs to be made on the specific German response to public health measures in American cities, and attempts need to be made to tie their seeming resistance to German medical thought of the period, to different waves of immigration, or to cultural habits. For a similar observation about German resistance to vaccination, see Martin Kaufman, "The American Anti-Vaccinationists and Their Arguments," *Bulletin of the History of Medicine* 41 (1967): 463–78.

14 I used the Pearson product moment correlation r. The 1890 correlation was $+.65$ and tested significant at the $p < .01$ level; the 1900, $+.50$, significant at $< .05$. Interestingly, a similar correlation drawn for 1910 did not offer a high correlation $(+.18)$, possibly indicating that density in housing was losing importance in a period when medical acumen, hospital facilities, and availability of medical care were increasing. Density per dwelling was more reliable than density per ward because in many parts of the city empty space still existed in wards, such as the fourteenth, that were otherwise congested.

15 Wisconsin State Board of Health, *Sixth Annual Report, 1881* (Madison, 1882), p. 112.

16 Wisconsin State Board of Health, *Seventh Annual Report, 1882* (Madison, 1883), pp. 234–35.

17 City of Madison, *Board of Health Report* (Madison: Democrat Printing Co., 1885), p. 1.

18 Wisconsin State Board of Health, *Ninth Annual Report, 1885* (Madison, 1886), p. 105.

19 Ibid., p. 171.

20 MHD, *Fourth Annual Report* (1871), p. 39.

21 E. S. Chesbrough, *Report on Milwaukee Water Works, Submitted by E. S. Chesbrough, Civil Engineer, to His Honor the Mayor and the Committee on Water Works of the City of Milwaukee, October 28, 1868* (Milwaukee: Daily News Steam Book and Job Print, 1868). Copy in the library of the State Historical Society of Wisconsin, Madison, Wis. For more on Chesbrough, see Louis P. Cain, "Raising and Watering a City: Ellis Sylvester Chesbrough and Chicago's First Sanitation System," *Technology and Culture* 13 (1972): 353–72.

22 MHD, *Tenth Annual Report* (1876), p. 68.

23 Laurence M. Larson, *A Financial and Administrative History of Milwaukee* (Madison: Wisconsin State Historical Society, 1908), p. 111. For more on

Milwaukee's water mains, see the Milwaukee Board of Public Works annual reports and Samuel Weidman and Alfred Schultz, *The Underground and Surface Water Supplies of Wisconsin*, Wisconsin Geological and Natural History Survey, 35, Economic Series No. 17 (Madison: published by the State, 1915), pp. 454–57.

24 *Evening Wisconsin* (Milwaukee), July 29, 1879.

25 Milwaukee *Daily News*, August 28, 1879.

26 MHD, *Thirty-Fifth Annual Report* (1911), p. 94.

27 Milwaukee *State Journal and South Side Advocate*, July 10, 1879; U.O.B. Wingate, in communication to the common council, *Proceedings of the Common Council of the City of Milwaukee for the Year Ending April 20th, 1891* (Milwaukee: Ed. Keogh, 1891), September 8, 1890, p. 354.

28 MHD, *Eighth Annual Report* (1875), p. 34.

29 Milwaukee *Sentinel*, June 29, 1887.

30 MHD, *Twelfth Annual Report* (1878), p. 88.

31 Ibid., p. 85. For more on the impact of sewer gas on sanitarians in this period, see Deanna Reed Springall, "The Sewer Gas Theory of Disease: A Period of Transition in Medical Etiology" (Master's thesis, University of Wisconsin, Madison, 1977).

32 Robert Martin, "Disposal of Garbage at Milwaukee," *Public Health: Papers and Reports of the APHA* 15 (1889): 64.

33 Milwaukee *Sentinel*, January 22, 1869, p. 1.

34 For the specific figures in the years 1867 to 1910 see MHD, *Thirty-Third Annual Report* (1909), pp. 37–38. For a lengthy discussion of Milwaukee's experience with garbage, see Leavitt, "Public Health in Milwaukee," pp. 182–250.

35 MHD, *Thirty-Third Annual Report*, p. 13.

36 MHD, *Eighth Annual Report*, pp. 8–9; and Milwaukee *Sentinel*, April 6, 1907.

37 O. W. Wight, quoted in the Milwaukee *Sentinel*, December 30, 1882.

38 Dr. Edward Evans, speaking during the discussion of J. M. Furstman, "A City Health Department," *Wisconsin Medical Journal* 11 (1912–13): 149–52.

39 Caution must be used in attributing infant mortality drops to improvements in the milk supply. It is no doubt true that cleaning the milk aided infant and child health, but it is impossible to determine how many and what age children drank cow's milk, and therefore a direct cause and effect relationship cannot be determined.

40 Milwaukee *Sentinel*, December 18, 1894; MHD, *Eighteenth Annual Report* (1895), pp. 8–9; MHD, *Eighteenth and Nineteenth Annual Report* (1896), p. 19.

41 Furstman, "City Health Department," pp. 149–52.

42 For an example of how politics can influence and complicate a health issue, see Judith W. Leavitt, "Politics and Public Health: Smallpox in Milwaukee, 1894–1895," *Bulletin of the History of Medicine* 50 (1976): 553–68.

43 These figures were derived from *Polk's Medical and Surgical Register of the United States and Canada* (Chicago: R. L. Polk and Co., 1900).

44 S. J. Crumbine, "Health Progress in Wisconsin Cities," *Wisconsin Medical Journal* 24 (1925): 360–69.

45 See William Butterworth, "Inter-Chamber Health Conservation Contest," *American Journal of Public Health* 20 (1930): 635. See also George A. Dundon, "Health Chronology of Milwaukee," undated typescript, copy in the Milwaukee Health Department library; and miscellaneous clippings in the Milwaukee Health Department library.

8 *Ronald L. Numbers*

A Note on Medical Education in Wisconsin

Wisconsin offered virtually no formal training in medicine until the 1890s.[1] Until then many aspiring physicians, especially in the early days, simply learned medicine on the job while serving as apprentices to local practitioners. Those desiring medical degrees traveled to Chicago or beyond to enroll in a medical school. Although some medical schools had university or other institutional connections, more were run by private individuals for prestige or profit. Well into the second half of the nineteenth century, both university and proprietary schools required little more of M.D. candidates than attendance at two identical lecture courses of about three months' duration. The four-year graded curriculum did not appear until late in the century.[2]

Whatever the reasons for Wisconsin's slowness in acquiring a medical school, the legislature bears no blame. In 1848 the new state's lawmakers called for the creation of a university in Madison comprising four departments: law; medicine; the theory and practice of elementary instruction; and science, literature and the arts. Legislators subsequently granted charters to several private concerns. But for decades all attempts to establish a viable medical school ended in failure, and sixty years passed before the University of Wisconsin took advantage of the 1848 law and opened a two-year medical school.

Following an abortive attempt by several Milwaukee physicians to

177

organize a medical school under the university's charter, the Board of Regents of the University of Wisconsin in 1854 voted to establish a medical department in Madison. Within two years the board had filled seven professorships, appointed a dean, and announced the beginning of classes for the spring of 1858. When the time came to admit students, however, the intended home of the medical department (present-day Bascom Hall) remained unfinished, and the board postponed the opening — for fifty years.

After the Civil War, Milwaukee physicians tried twice again to capture the medical department for their city, but each time they returned from Madison empty-handed. In 1875 University President John Bascom proposed the creation of a medical branch of the university in Milwaukee, which afforded "far more clinical advantages than Madison," but the state medical society blocked the plan after learning of Bascom's intention to grant "equal privileges to all systems of Medicine," sectarian as well as regular. For the remainder of the century the state's regular physicians expressed little enthusiasm for the prospect of competing with well-trained graduates from the state university in an already overcrowded profession.

The state medical society did, however, support the creation in 1887 of a premedical course, which allowed Wisconsin students to save a year when they enrolled in one of the three Chicago medical schools. Initially, Edward A. Birge, a biologist, taught all of the required premedical subjects: zoology, vertebrate anatomy, histology, physiology, and bacteriology. The program proved so successful that the university in 1892 added a second instructor, William Snow Miller, who had studied with Franklin P. Mall, the nation's foremost anatomist. Twelve years later the university recruited a second student of Mall's, Charles R. Bardeen, who came from Johns Hopkins to lay the groundwork for a two-year medical school.

Perhaps shamed by the realization that the neighboring state universities of Michigan, Illinois, Iowa, and Minnesota already supported complete four-year medical schools, the legislature in 1907 voted to establish a half-school at Madison that would offer two years of instruction in the preclinical sciences. Bardeen, who became dean of the new school, immediately began hiring the best young faculty he could find, especially among Hopkins alumni. One of his earliest recruits, Joseph Erlanger, later won a Nobel prize, and others went on to distinguished careers. Working out of attic laboratories in Science Hall, Bardeen and his young colleagues soon created what may have been the strongest half-school in the country.

During the six decades it took the University of Wisconsin to make up

its mind about medical education, there were a number of attempts —
mostly unsuccessful — to fill the state's medical-school vacuum. As early
as 1848 one enterprising group of physicians won legislative approval
for a Madison Medical College and "a branch of the same." Ignoring
Madison, the incorporators opened a "branch" in northern Illinois under the name of Rock Island Medical College, which appears to have
been their original goal. After only one course of lectures the peripatetic
branch moved on to Davenport, Iowa, and still later to Keokuk. Following the move to Iowa, one of the Wisconsin founders, Chandler B.
Chapman, briefly offered private "Instruction in Anatomy and Practical Surgery" in some dissecting rooms on State Street in Madison, but no
Madison Medical College ever appeared.

On the eve of the Civil War the La Crosse County Medical Society
talked the trustees of Galesville University in nearby Trempealeau
County into sponsoring a medical department in La Crosse. Little came
of the scheme besides the temporary appointment of one William M.
Young to a professorship in the department. In 1864, however, the state
legislature granted a charter for an independent La Crosse Medical
College. Although the trustees met annually until the early 1880s, and a
faculty existed on paper, no students ever enrolled. Occasionally the

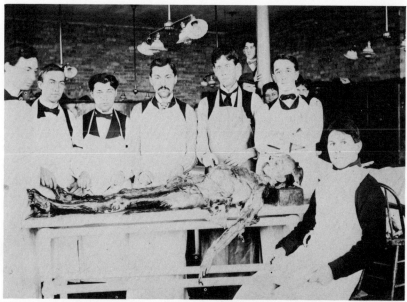

State Historical Society of Wisconsin, WHi(X3)26037

A group of medical students studying human anatomy.

"professors" lectured to one another or performed a dissection for their own edification.

Milwaukee, with a population much larger than Madison or La Crosse, has the dubious honor of being the home of the state's first functioning medical school. Although Milwaukee physicians in 1848 received a charter for a Wisconsin Medical College and tried for decades to obtain the University of Wisconsin's medical department, no medical school appeared until 1881, when William H. Coney and friends organized the Milwaukee College of Physicians and Surgeons, known locally as the Coney Medical Institute. Coney, a former "coal heaver at the gasworks," claimed to be an M.D., but he almost certainly never attended medical school. After operating "some sort of a hot bath concern" in downtown Milwaukee for a while, he decided in 1881 to turn it into a medical school. According to one newspaper, students could obtain an M.D. from the Coney Medical Institute in no more than ten hours: "Walking in at 7 o'clock, the applicant could hear the lectures, make his studies, pass an examination, and leave the institution in the evening a regular practitioner, with diploma, certificate, and the necessary appurtenances."[3] Diplomas could also be purchased outright. In September 1883, the Milwaukee health commissioner, accompanied by several prominent physicians, inspected the institute. Anticipating a negative report, Coney voluntarily shut down what had apparently become a lucrative business.

Degree mills reappeared in Milwaukee in the 1890s. The Wisconsin Eclectic Medical College, which opened in 1894 and graduated its only class in 1896, embarrassed even the sectarians — especially after its dean was arrested for selling diplomas. In 1896 the attorney general also closed down Milwaukee University for fraudulently selling medical diplomas for two hundred dollars. By comparison, the Milwaukee Institute of Osteopathy, which survived for three years, looks almost respectable, even though its academic credentials were marginal at best (see Chapter 3 in this volume).

The first medical school in the state worthy of the name, the Wisconsin College of Physicians and Surgeons, opened in Milwaukee in 1893 with 42 students. Initially organized as a joint-stock company, the school in 1906 abandoned efforts to make money and subsequently became a member of the Association of American Medical Colleges. Although run independently, it operated nominally as the medical department of Carroll College.

Within a year of its founding the Wisconsin College of Physicians and Surgeons faced competition from a second regular medical school, the

WISCONSIN COLLEGE

OF

PHYSICIANS and SURGEONS

(Opposite St. Joseph's Hospital)

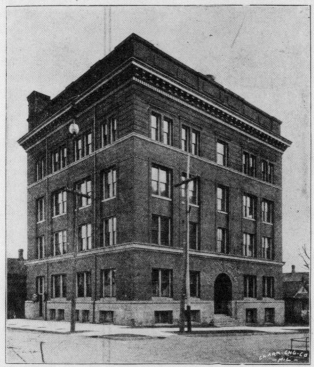

Co-Educational DEPARTMENT OF MEDICINE
DEPARTMENT OF DENTISTRY

The Annual Session begins
about October 1st each year
and continues eight months

Standard requirements for admission. ⁊ Laboratory facilities unexcelled. ⁊ Clinical advantages ample. Fees moderate. | Persons interested in Medical or Dental education are invited to investigate this school.

JAS. T. STUART, D.D.S., Dean of Dental Dept., 31 Pierce Bldg.
W. H. WASHBURN, M.D., Secretary, 1240 Wells Building.

Wisconsin Medical Journal 2 (1903–4): xxii

The Wisconsin College of Physicians and Surgeons, founded in Milwaukee in 1893 as the medical department of Carroll College, was the state's first regular medical school. In 1913 Marquette University adopted it as its School of Medicine.

Milwaukee Medical College and School of Dentistry, also a joint-stock company. During its early history this institution engaged in practices so questionable that the Milwaukee County Medical Society in 1902 called it "a menace to the reputation and good standing of the medical profession of the city and state." The next year the Association of American Medical Colleges "severely censured" it. Nevertheless, Marquette University in 1907 adopted the Milwaukee Medical College as its medical department.

When Abraham Flexner inspected the two Milwaukee schools in February 1910, he found a dismal situation. The Milwaukee Medical College, with 168 students and 67 instructors, had "meager" laboratory facilities, except for anatomy, and "extremely weak" clinical facilities. The Wisconsin College of Physicians and Surgeons, with an enrollment of 60 and a teaching staff of 66, all part-time, occupied an attractive but poorly equipped building containing

an ordinary laboratory for elementary chemistry, another — poor and very disorderly, without animals — for bacteriology; the room given to histology and pathology is clean, contains a small amount of well kept material, and is adequate to routine elementary work. Anatomy is very poor; there is not even a complete skeleton. No other teaching adjuncts are at hand. No provision is made for even demonstrative work in experimental physiology.

The clinical facilities Flexner described as "utterly wretched." The two Milwaukee schools, he concluded in his final report, "are without a redeeming feature."[4]

Two years after the publication of Flexner's survey, conditions in Milwaukee remained so bad that the American Medical Association's Council on Medical Education threatened both schools with a "C" rating, the lowest possible. Aroused students at the Milwaukee Medical College responded with a mass meeting, demanding that the school undertake immediate reforms. When the administration failed to act, "the entire student body left the Milwaukee Medical College and marched to the Wisconsin College of Physicians and Surgeons and enrolled themselves there with the understanding that action would be taken" to ensure a decent rating.[5] Bereft of its students, the Milwaukee Medical College passed away — freeing Marquette University from what had become an embarrassing relationship.

At the urging of local physicians, Marquette in 1913 purchased the financially plagued Wisconsin College of Physicians and Surgeons and leased the physical remains of the Milwaukee Medical College. Under the leadership of Dean Louis J. Jermain, the resulting Marquette University School of Medicine within two years received an "A" grade from the Council on Medical Education. Aided by wartime patriotism and a grant of $333,333 from the Carnegie Foundation, the Marquette school by the close of the decade had raised an endowment of one million dollars. But just as the school seemed headed for a bright future, a bitter public quarrel between the university's Jesuit fathers and the medical staff over therapeutic abortions led to the resignations of many of the most prominent faculty members. Once again Jermain rebuilt the faculty to respectability, remaining as dean until 1926. Four decades later the school, in need of state funds, severed its relations with Marquette, and in 1970 it changed its name to the Medical College of Wisconsin.

In contrast to the dismal facilities he discovered in Milwaukee, Flexner found the University of Wisconsin's half-school to be a model of its kind. Unlike the Milwaukee institutions, which paid only lip service to a high-school diploma entrance requirement, the Madison faculty "rigidly enforced" its rule of two years of previous college work. Seventeen of the 23 instructors taught full-time and occupied laboratories "admirably equipped with respect to both teaching and research," though poorly located. The school lacked only a new building.[6]

Flexner anticipated the day when the Madison school would expand its two-year curriculum into a complete course, and he urged that this be done in Madison rather than Milwaukee. Dean Bardeen agreed, arguing that "no expenditure of public funds is likely to give greater return than that spent for scientific treatment of disease." Appealing to regional rivalry, he pointed out that the bordering states of Michigan, Illinois, Iowa, and Minnesota already had complete medical departments at their universities, leaving Wisconsin "far behind" in the field of medical education. Besides, he said, Wisconsin lost its best young physicians by sending them out of state to complete their training. Swayed by such arguments, the legislature in 1919 approved the creation of a four-year medical course at Madison.

To obtain the necessary teaching hospital, the governor took money from the soldiers' bonus fund and built Wisconsin General Hospital as a memorial to the veterans of the First World War. The staff of the Student Health Service, begun in 1910, became the core of the clinical faculty. In addition, Bardeen lined up physicians from around the state to serve as preceptors, thus providing Wisconsin's students with practical experience similar to the nineteenth-century apprenticeship. In 1925 the medical school admitted its first clinical students and two years later awarded its first M.D.s to a class of 19 men and 6 women.

When Bardeen retired as dean in 1935, he turned over a thriving medical school to William S. Middleton, a distinguished clinician who had been with the university since 1912. During his two decades as dean, Middleton built outstanding programs in such diverse areas as cancer research and medical history. Study of the history of medicine had flourished in Madison since 1909, when William Snow Miller began his famous seminars, but until 1947 and the appointment of Erwin H. Ackerknecht as professor of the history of medicine, the subject lacked formal recognition. With the creation of a permanent department three years later, Wisconsin became the second American university (after Johns Hopkins) to so recognize the subject.[7]

Throughout the twentieth century, Wisconsin's two medical schools have supplied the state with well-trained physicians, general practitioners as well as specialists. If neither school ranks among the nation's leaders in medical education, at least both are far from the bottom. A poll of medical educators, published in 1977, listed the University of Wisconsin School of Medicine twenty-eighth in "perceived quality" among 94 medical schools in the United States. It still lagged behind Michigan (no. 8) and Minnesota (no. 12), but Dean Bardeen would have been proud to see that Wisconsin no longer trailed Iowa (no. 32) and Illinois (no. 39). The Medical College of Wisconsin tied for fifty-sixth place.[8]

Notes

1 This chapter's account of medical education in Wisconsin is based largely on Paul F. Clark, *The University of Wisconsin Medical School: A Chronicle, 1848–1948* (Madison: University of Wisconsin Press, for the Wisconsin Medical Alumni Association, 1967); Raphael N. Hamilton, *The Story of Marquette University* (Milwaukee: Marquette University Press, 1953); William Snow Miller, "The La Crosse Medical School," *Wisconsin Medical Journal* 33 (1934): 11–23; William Snow Miller, "Medical Schools in Wisconsin: Past and Present," *Wisconsin Medical Journal* 35 (1936): 472–86; G. Kasten Tallmadge, "Medical Education in Milwaukee, 1848–1893," *Wisconsin Medical Journal* 36 (1937): 303–16; William S. Middleton, "The First Medical Faculty of the University of Wisconsin," *Wisconsin Medical Journal* 54 (1955): 378–85, 428–38; and Walter Zeit, "Marquette University School of Medicine: The First Fifty Years," *Wisconsin Medical Journal* 62 (1963): 295–302.

2 See Ronald L. Numbers, ed., *The Education of American Physicians: Historical Essays* (Berkeley: University of California Press, 1980).

3 Tallmadge, "Medical Education in Milwaukee," pp. 308, 310.

4 Abraham Flexner, *Medical Education in the United States and Canada* (New York: Carnegie Foundation, 1910), pp. 317–19.

5 Hamilton, *The Story of Marquette University*, p. 75.

6 Flexner, *Medical Education*, pp. 317–19.

7 Guenter B. Risse, "An Account of the Wisconsin Chair in Medical History: A Tribute to William S. Middleton," *Bulletin of the History of Medicine* 50 (1976): 133–37.

8 Jonathan R. Cole and James A. Lipton, "The Reputations of American Medical Schools," *Social Forces* 55 (1977): 662–84.

Deanna Reed Springall

Selected Sources
on the History of Medicine
in Wisconsin

This bibliography is intended to serve as an introduction both to previous research on the history of medicine in Wisconsin and to the resources available for future research. It is not a comprehensive listing of
all sources, but simply a sampling of the great variety of manuscripts
and publications covering Wisconsin's medical history in the nineteenth
and twentieth centuries.

Primary Sources

The primary sources listed below are housed in the Middleton Medical Library (MML) at the University of Wisconsin–Madison; the State
Historical Society of Wisconsin (SHSW), in Madison; the Area Research
Center (ARC) at the University of Wisconsin–Milwaukee; the Milwaukee Academy of Medicine (MAM), and the Legislative Reference Bureau (LRB) in Milwaukee. The State Historical Society also maintains
one of the nation's largest newspaper collections (second only to the
Library of Congress), including numerous nineteenth-century Wisconsin newspapers.

Medical Publications

Bulletin of the Wisconsin State Nurses Association, 1933–1956; *STAT!*
1957–present. MML

A periodical from the Wisconsin State Nurses Association.

Homeopathic Expositor, 1866–1868. MML
A short-lived publication by the homeopathic physicians of Milwaukee which advanced the merits of their medical beliefs.

Marquette Medical Review, 1936–1969. MML
A journal published by the students of the Marquette University School of Medicine. It included many clinical presentations, but also provided an "outlet for student expression relative to recent advances in medicine."

Milwaukee Homeopathic Medical Reporter, 1848. SHSW (Microfilm)
A monthly volume published between January and December, 1848.

Milwaukee Medical Journal, 1893–1912. MML
A "monthly journal of medicine and surgery," devoted to the entire profession and not to any particular individuals or sects.

Milwaukee Medical Times, 1928–1956; *Milwaukee Medical Society Times*, 1956–present. MML
A publication of the Medical Society of Milwaukee County. The *Times* includes many articles on medical history over the years.

Proceedings of the Wisconsin State Medical Society, 1855, 1856; *Transactions of the State Medical Society of Wisconsin*, 1869–1902. MML
Reports of the officers, addresses of the presidents, contributed papers, and lists of officers and members. Publication was continued in the *Wisconsin Medical Journal* after 1902.

Wisconsin Dental Review, 1925–1939; *Journal of the Wisconsin State Dental Society*, 1940–1973; *Journal of the Wisconsin Dental Association*, 1974–present. MML
A publication of the Wisconsin Dental Association. Editorials and scientific articles are included, as well as reports from the annual meetings.

Wisconsin Medical Alumni Journal, May 1956–?; *Wisconsin Medical Alumni Newsletter*, ?–Fall 1962; *Wisconsin Medical Alumni Bulletin*, Winter 1963–Spring 1965; *Wisconsin Medical Alumni Quarterly*, Summer 1965–present. MML
A periodical from the Wisconsin Medical Alumni Association. Many articles describe events at the University of Wisconsin School of Medicine.

Wisconsin Medical Journal, 1903–present. MML
The official publication of the State Medical Society of Wisconsin. Editorials and presidential addresses are an excellent source of medical opinion; scientific articles reveal much about the state of medical practice. One issue per year (since 1925) is the "Medical Blue Book," which summarizes the rules and regulations affecting physicians in

their practice. The *Journal* frequently includes articles on medical history.

Wisconsin Medical Recorder, 1898–1915. MML
A "monthly journal of medicine and surgery for the whole profession."

Wisconsin Osteopath, 1898–1900. MML
A journal which proposed to "introduce, explain and advance the new science." It was published by the Milwaukee Institute of Osteopathy, August 1898–March 1899; by the Milwaukee College of Osteopathy, April 1899–August 1900.

Boards of Health, Reports and Bulletins

Green Bay. Board of Health, *Annual Report*, 1894–present. SHSW

Madison. Board of Health, *Report*, 1885–1943. Health Department, *Report*, 1944–1946. Department of Public Health, *Report*, 1947–1949. Health Department, *Report*, 1950. Department of Public Health, *Report*, 1951–present. SHSW

Milwaukee. Health Department, *Annual Report*, 1868–present. LRB, SHSW

Milwaukee. Health Department, *Bulletin*, 1911; *The Healthologist*, 1911–1914; *Bulletin*, 1915–1942. SHSW

Milwaukee. Health Department, *Monthly Report – Summary of Statistics*, 1886–1910. SHSW

Racine. Health Department, *Annual Report*, 1884–1950; *Annual Statistical Report*, 1951–present. SHSW

Wisconsin. State Board of Health, *Annual Report*, 1876–1882; *Report*, 1882/84–1946/47; *Biennial Report*, 1948/50–1964/66. MML, SHSW

Wisconsin. State Board of Health, *Annual Report of Morbidity and Mortality*, 1948; *Morbidity and Mortality*, 1949–1951; *Public Health Statistics*, 1952–1965. Division of Health, *Public Health Statistics*, 1966–present. SHSW

Wisconsin. State Board of Health, *Bulletin*, 1904–1940; *Quarterly Bulletin*, 1940–1948; *Bimonthly Bulletin*, 1948; *Health*, 1949–1967. Division of Health, *Health*, 1968; *Wisconsin's Health*, 1969–1975; *Health in Wisconsin*, 1976–present. MML, SHSW

Manuscripts and Documents: Medical Associations

Ashland-Bayfield-Iron County Medical Society. Minutes, 1903–1948. SHSW

Ashland Medical Society. Records, 1892, including constitution, by-laws and a fee schedule. SHSW

Bartlett Clinical Club (also known as The Clinical Club). Minutes, papers, and correspondence, 1886–1891. MAM

Brown County Medical Society. Minute book, including financial and treasurers' reports, 1903–1927. SHSW

Brown–Kewaunee–Door County Medical Society. Minimum fee schedules, 1906, c. 1918, and 1937. SHSW

Dane County Medical Society (also known as the Wisconsin Central Medical Association and the Central Wisconsin Medical Association). Minutes and ledgers, 1850–1917. State Medical Society of Wisconsin, Madison.

Dodge County Medical Society. Papers, 1905–1948, containing monthly newsletters, minute books, society correspondence, and letters from Army surgeons in the Second World War. Minutes, 1894–1937. SHSW

Eau Claire–Dunn–Pepin County Medical Society. Minutes, 1934–1946. SHSW

Fee schedule adopted in 1844 by the physicians of Milwaukee. SHSW

Fee schedule adopted in 1879 by the physicians and surgeons of Beloit. SHSW

Fee schedule adopted by the physicians and surgeons of Waukesha in the early 1890s. SHSW

Fond du Lac County Medical Society. Papers, 1868–1876, 1902–1935, containing minute books, membership lists, papers read before the society, an early constitution, fee schedules, and some incoming correspondence. SHSW

Fox River Valley Medical Society. Records and minutes, 1886–1926. SHSW

Homeopathic Medical Society of the State of Wisconsin. Minutes, 1865–1910, 1927–1953. SHSW

Jefferson County Medical Society. Records, 1903–1945, consisting of minutes, treasurers' records, resolutions, and papers. SHSW

Lincoln County Medical Society. Minute book, 1903–1938, including constitution and minutes (1893–1894) of the Merrill Physicians Protective Association. SHSW

Marathon County Medical Society. Minute book, 1903–1934. SHSW

Medico-Chirurgical Club. Records, 1851–1853. MAM

Milwaukee Academy of Medicine. Correspondence, 1904–1916. MAM

Milwaukee City Medical Association. Minutes, papers and correspondence, 1847–1880. MAM

Milwaukee County Medical Society. Minute book, 1846–1879, constitution, bylaws, and list of original members. SHSW

Milwaukee Medical Society (also known as the Medical and Surgical Club). Minutes, papers and correspondence, 1869–1872, 1876–1880, 1891–1905. MAM

Northwestern Wisconsin Medical Association. Ninth Councilor District Medical Society. Records, 1879–1930, consisting of a minute book, constitution and bylaws, limited correspondence, and announcements of the association's meetings, 1928–1930. SHSW

Portage County Medical Society. Minute book, 1903–1937. SHSW

Prairie du Chien area. Papers, 1809–1847, relating to the area around Prairie du Chien, including medical records from Fort Crawford. SHSW

Waukesha County Medical Society. Papers (1842–1920) including early records and officers' names, minute book (1911–1921), membership lists, constitution, and bylaws. SHSW

Winnebago County Medical Society. Records and minutes, 1865–1897. SHSW

Wisconsin Anti-Tuberculosis Association. Papers, 1908–1930, consisting of reports and speeches on tuberculosis. SHSW

Wisconsin Nurses Association, Milwaukee District. Records, 1928–1954, including minutes, correspondence, and reports. ARC

Wisconsin State Eclectic Medical Society. Records, containing minutes (1901–1934), ledger book (1893–1908), account book (1909–1934), constitution, and bylaws. SHSW

Manuscripts and Documents: Physicians' Records

Belitz, Alfred. Papers, 1897–1951, of a Pepin physician, including correspondence, 1909–1951; unpublished manuscripts, speeches, and articles; biographical material; and several volumes listing daily calls. SHSW

Brays, William H. Formula book, 1862–1864, including numerous medical recipes. SHSW

Brown, I. M. Notebook (c. 1898) of a New London physician pertaining to infant care. SHSW

Chapman, Chandler Burnell. Papers, 1835–1901, of a Madison physician and surgeon. SHSW

Coumbe, Warner R. Records, 1901–1908, 1919–1920, of a Richland Center physician, consisting of patients' accounts, case histories, prescriptions, and fees. SHSW

Dodd, John M. Papers, 1881–1920, of an Ashland physician, consisting of correspondence, 1881–1899; case histories and account books, 1889–1907; and notes on medical practice. SHSW

Doughty, Perry W. Ledgers, 1908–1922, of an Eau Galle physician, in-

cluding medical charges and drug costs. Some of these costs were incurred during the 1918 influenza epidemic. SHSW

Fox, William H., and Fox, Philip. Account ledgers, 1864–1871, of two
physicians who practiced in and around Oregon. SHSW

Gregory, Levi M. Account ledger, 1850–1851, of a physician who practiced in Plover. SHSW

Harper, Cornelius A. Papers, 1875–1891, 1905–1915, 1922–1929, 1944,
including information on the early years of the Wisconsin State Board
of Health and biographical material on the board members. SHSW

Hoyt, Ralph G. Account books, 1861–1916, of a Menomonee Falls physician and of his parents, both practicing physicians. ARC

Hurlbut, John Albert. Papers, 1918–1958, of an ear, nose, and throat
specialist at Madison's Jackson Clinic. SHSW

Kleinpell, Henry. Papers, 1918–1951, including medical notebooks, records and correspondence from his Prairie du Chien practice. SHSW

Kosanke, Frederic E. Papers, 1900–1954, of a Fond du Lac homeopathic practitioner, consisting of correspondence, 1929–1954, a ledger, 1900–1952, and a cash book, 1906–1953. His letters from 1931 to
1932 discussed the conflict between the state Homeopathic Medical
Society and the State Medical Society of Wisconsin over membership
on the Wisconsin State Board of Medical Examiners. SHSW

LaCount, David. Account books and ledgers, 1858–1892, of a Chilton
practitioner. SHSW

Loy, William. Daybook, 1882–1896, of a Platteville physician. SHSW

Malcolm, W. G. Records, 1898–1936, of a Chetek physician including
daybooks, ledgers of medical accounts receivable, records of narcotic
drugs dispensed, and correspondence. SHSW

Manley, Ira. Papers, 1860–1892, of a Markesan physician who was assistant surgeon of the First Wisconsin Heavy Artillery during the
Civil War. SHSW

Miller, B. O. Accounts for medical attendance at Prairie du Chien,
1834–1835, 1837–1838. SHSW

Munk, Emanuel. Papers, 1861–1893, of a German-American physician
who practiced in Fond du Lac and Milwaukee, including Civil War
correspondence and letters. SHSW

Reeve, James Theodore. Diary, October 1864–December 1865, of a surgeon, Twenty-First Regiment, Wisconsin Volunteers. SHSW

Reynolds, B. O. Correspondence and speeches, 1878–1881, chiefly discussing the licensing law for doctors introduced in the 1878–1879 session of the state legislature. SHSW

Sawtell, Price. Medical recipes of a doctor who began practice near
Milwaukee in 1848. SHSW

Schein, John E. Papers, 1905–1948, of an Oshkosh physician, consisting of office records and accounts; record books of Metropolitan Life Insurance Company cases, 1937–1940; South Side Hospital ledger, 1918–1921; and a daybook, 1921. SHSW

Schreiner, Johan K. Daybooks, 1884, 1886–1889, of a Westby physician, with patients' names, charges, and services rendered. SHSW

Trautmann, Milton. Papers, 1932–1963, of a Prairie du Sac physician, including appointments, charges, treatments, receipts and expenditures, inoculations, obstetrical cases, and records of narcotic drugs dispensed. SHSW

Youmans, John B. Records, 1846–1883, of a Mukwonago physician, including daybooks and ledgers. ARC

Secondary and Other Sources

Much of the medical history of Wisconsin has appeared in the form of reminiscences and biographies of physicians and in histories of medical institutions and organizations. Many of the sources listed below include further references.

Medical Personnel and Their Practice

Alexander, Edward P. "Surgeon Beaumont at Prairie du Chien." *Wisconsin Medical Journal* 44 (October 1945): 1006–1009.

A description of the famous experiments in gastric physiology which William Beaumont conducted at Fort Crawford in the 1820s and 1830s. Though much has been written about Beaumont, this article and the one by Connors deal specifically with Beaumont's Wisconsin experiences.

Apple, Rima D., and Leavitt, Judith Walzer. "Women at the University of Wisconsin Medical School." In *University Women: A Series of Essays*, Vol. 2, *Wisconsin Women, Graduate School, and the Professions*, edited by Marian J. Swoboda and Audrey J. Roberts. Madison: UW Office of Women, 1980, pp. 55–64.

A statistical review and discussion of the role of women students and staff at the University of Wisconsin School of Medicine since its preclinical program began in 1907.

Bossard, Marcus. *Eighty-One Years of Living.* Minneapolis: Midwest Printing Co., 1946.

The medical practice of a Wisconsin-born physician. Bossard located in Spring Green in 1887 and practiced there most of his life. He drew particular attention to his introduction of surgical asepsis in the community.

Bradford, Thomas L. "Homoeopathy in Wisconsin." In *History of Homoeopathy and Its Institutions in America*, edited by William H. King. 4 vols. New York: The Lewis Publishing Company, 1905. 1:337–41.
The beginnings of homeopathy in Wisconsin, including the formation of three different state societies in 1848, 1858, and 1865.

Bull, James. "The First Experimental Surgical Laboratory in Milwaukee." *Marquette Medical Review* 32 (Winter 1966): 17–18.
A summary of the experiments conducted in the late 1800s at the animal research laboratory of Nicholas Senn.

Bultena, Gordon L. "The Changing Distribution and Adequacy of Medical, Dental and Hospital Services in Rural and Urban Communities in Wisconsin, 1910–1960." Madison: University of Wisconsin, Department of Rural Sociology, 1966.
Documentation on the declining availability of health services in rural Wisconsin communities.

Burke, Fred D. "Recollections of Early Day Medical Practice in a Saw Mill Village."
A manuscript in the State Historical Society of Wisconsin.

Campenni, Frank J. *History of Dentistry in Wisconsin*. Milwaukee(?): Wisconsin State Dental Society, 1970.
A reprinting of a series of historical articles from the *Journal of the Wisconsin State Dental Society* in commemoration of the society's centennial (1870–1970).

Connors, Dean M. "William Beaumont, M.D.: A Wisconsin Legacy." *Wisconsin Medical Journal* 76 (October 1977): 22–26.
An overview of Beaumont's medical practice, including his interests in vaccination, malaria, and cholera.

Cooper, Signe S. *Wisconsin Nursing Pioneers*. Madison: University Extension, University of Wisconsin, 1968.
Brief biographies of the early nursing leaders in Wisconsin.

Custer, G. Stanley. "The Development of Group Practice in the Midwest and Wisconsin." *Wisconsin Medical Journal* 75 (July 1976): 32–37.
Descriptions of the origins of several clinics both in the Midwest and in Wisconsin.

Davenport, F. Garvin, and Davenport, Katye Lou, eds. "Practicing Medicine in Madison, 1855–57: Alexander Schue's Letters to Robert Peter." *Wisconsin Magazine of History* 26 (1942–43): 79–91.
Letters from a Madison physician to a Transylvania University chemist, including some references to medical practice in Madison.

Dodd, John M. *Autobiography of a Surgeon*. New York: Walter Neale, 1928.

The life and practice of a Pennsylvania-born physician who practiced in Wausau, Rhinelander, and Ashland in the late nineteenth and early twentieth centuries. Half of the book describes his childhood, medical education, and practice; the second half is a collection of papers on surgical procedures, medical treatment, and medical thought.

Falk, Victor S. "Wisconsin's Surgical Heritage." *Wisconsin Medical Journal* 75 (April 1976): 24–28.
Brief biographies of some of Wisconsin's early surgeons.

Frank, Louis Frederick. *Medical History of Milwaukee, 1834–1914.* Milwaukee: Germania Publishing Co., 1915.
A thorough compilation of facts about Milwaukee's medical history. Most of the book is devoted to biographies, vital statistics, and historical sketches of medical societies and hospitals.

Habbe, J. E. "Milwaukee's Radiologic Heritage." *Wisconsin Medical Journal* 64 (March 1965): 125–29.
A description of the early use of X-rays in Milwaukee and the founding and activities of the Milwaukee Roentgen Ray Society.

Hammond, F. W. "Seventy Years in the Practice of Medicine." Manitowoc County Historical Society, *Occupational Monograph 6*, 1968 Series, pp. 3–10.
The practice of a physician in Wyocena and Manitowoc in the early 1900s. Several common diseases and their treatments are described.

Harstad, Peter T., ed. "A Civil War Medical Examiner: The Report of Dr. Horace O. Crane." *Wisconsin Magazine of History* 48 (1964–65): 222–31.
The report of a surgeon who became one of Wisconsin's enrollment examiners during the Civil War. Crane mentions many of the frauds attempted by recruits who wished to avoid the draft.

Hebberd, Mary Hargrove. "Notes on Dr. David Franklin Powell, Known as 'White Beaver.'" *Wisconsin Magazine of History* 35 (1951–52): 306–309, and 36 (1952–53): 188–91.
The medical practice of a flamboyant La Crosse resident in the late nineteenth century. Powell's preferences for newspaper advertising and nostrums led to frequent clashes with his fellow practitioners.

Jenkins, G. W. "Reminiscences of Some Earlier Medical Practice in Wisconsin." *Wisconsin Medical Journal* 8 (March 1910): 549–56.
The experiences of a physician in Kilbourn from 1851 to 1906.

Johnson, F. G. "Experiences of a Pioneer Physician in Northern Wisconsin." *Wisconsin Medical Journal* 38 (July 1939): 576–88, and 38 (August 1939): 682–89.
The practice of a physician in lumbering and sawmill camps and towns in the early 1900s. The ticket system for hospitalization, early

efforts toward workmen's compensation and industrial insurance, and the influenza epidemic of 1918 are all included.

Kuhm, Herbert W. "Pioneer Dentistry in Wisconsin." *Wisconsin Magazine of History* 28 (1944–45): 154–68.
The early-nineteenth-century practice of several Wisconsin dentists.

McNeil, Donald R. "Dr. Alfred L. Castleman, Agitator and Critic." *Wisconsin Medical Journal* 51 (March 1952): 291–96.
The mid-nineteenth-century career of a controversial Wisconsin physician. Castleman pressed for the establishment of a state medical society, a state insane asylum, and a state medical school, and vigorously denounced all irregular practitioners. His short-lived political career was followed by Civil War service as an army surgeon.

Middleton, William S. "The First Medical Faculty at the University of Wisconsin." *Wisconsin Medical Journal* 54 (August 1955): 378–85, and 54 (September 1955): 428–38.
The efforts of Drs. Alfred L. Castleman, Ezra S. Carr, Joseph Hobbins, and Alexander Schue to establish a medical department at the University of Wisconsin in the 1850s.

Middleton, William S. "Howard Culbertson: Harvey Hospital Surgeon." *Wisconsin Medical Journal* 70 (November 1971): 47–52.
Events at a Madison Civil War hospital. Though not a Wisconsin resident, Culbertson served as the officer in charge of Harvey Hospital.

Munro, Jeanette. "Way Back When . . . : The First Perceptorship at Wisconsin." *Wisconsin Medical Alumni Quarterly* 18 (Winter 1978): 5–8.
A recollection of the three-month preceptorship of a Wisconsin medical student in La Crosse in 1927.

Phillips, Dennis H. "Women in Nineteenth Century Wisconsin Medicine." *Wisconsin Medical Journal* 71 (November 1972): 13–18.
Brief biographies of several nineteenth-century women physicians in Wisconsin.

"Reminiscences of Robert G. Sayle." *Wisconsin Medical Journal* 40 (August 1941): 747–51.
Events in the medical practice of a physician who located in Hales Corners and, later, Milwaukee, in the late 1800s and early 1900s. Several case histories are described.

Sargent, James W. "History of Urology in Wisconsin." *Wisconsin Medical Journal* 69 (July 1970): 182–86.
A summary of early work in urology by Wisconsin physicians. The founding of the Wisconsin Urological Society is also mentioned.

Shipman, Kirk W. "Osteopathy in Wisconsin, 1897 to 1940." A typescript in the State Historical Society of Wisconsin.

Washburn, William H. "Medical Practice in Wisconsin." *Wisconsin Medical Journal* 20 (December 1921): 324–28.

An overview of medical practice in the state from the mid-nineteenth to early twentieth century.

Organized Medicine

"An Epitome of the Development and Constructive Work of the State Medical Society of Wisconsin." *Wisconsin Medical Journal* 42 (January 1943): 26–53.

A chronological summary, 1841–1941, of the major accomplishments of Wisconsin's state medical society. Particular attention is devoted to the 1937–1938 studies on distribution of health service and sickness care in Wisconsin, the European system of compulsory sickness insurance, and voluntary systems of hospital insurance.

Evans, Curtis A. "Milwaukee Medical Societies: An Eighty-Five Year Retrospect." *Wisconsin Medical Journal* 22 (November 1923): 245–54.

Reviews and quotations from the minutes of several nineteenth-century Milwaukee medical societies.

Herriott, Marianne. "Placards and Pretenders: The Dane County Medical Society in the 'Good Old Days.'" *Wisconsin Medical Journal* 75 (October 1976): 14–16.

A description of some of the problems faced by Madison physicians and their medical society in the 1850s.

Miller, William Snow. "Dane County Medical Society." *Wisconsin Medical Journal* 36 (November 1937): 929–40, and 37 (July 1938): 580–94.

A detailed record of the activities of the Dane County Medical Society (also known as the Wisconsin Central Medical Association) from 1850 to 1870.

Miller, William Snow. "Early Efforts of the Wisconsin State Medical Society to Legalize Dissection." *Wisconsin Medical Journal* 34 (November 1935): 853–58.

The role of the state medical society in securing passage of an 1868 law to permit dissection.

Sivertson, Sigurd E. "The La Crosse County Medical Society." In *Phases of La Crosse County Medicine: 1855–1920.* La Crosse, Wis.: La Crosse County Medical Society, 1966.

A short history of a county medical society from 1855–1929, including an 1860 list of fees for surgery, house calls, and obstetrics.

"Specialty Section." *Milwaukee Medical Times*, May 1946, pp. 73–77.

Short histories of the Milwaukee Academy of Medicine and of specialty societies in surgery, oto-ophthalmology, radiology, internal medicine, pediatrics, gastroenterology, and neuropsychiatry.

Wisconsin State Medical Society, Woman's Auxiliary.

A review of the various nineteenth-century efforts to establish medical schools in Wisconsin.

"Nursing in Transition: Breaking Barriers of Tradition, 1924–1974." Bulletin of the University of Wisconsin, School of Nursing, Madison, 1974.
A short history of one of the oldest university nursing programs in the nation. Numerous photographs are included.

Robinson, Dale Wendell. *Wisconsin and the Mentally Ill: A History of the 'Wisconsin Plan' of State and County Care, 1860–1915.* New York: Arno Press, 1980.

Tallmadge, G. Kasten. "Medical Education in Milwaukee, 1848–1893." *Wisconsin Medical Journal* 36 (April 1937): 303–16.
A summary of the short-lived existence of several Milwaukee medical schools.

Triolo, Victor A. "The McArdle Story: Retrospect and Prospect." *Wisconsin Medical Alumni Newsletter* 4 (Fall 1964): 14–18.
A thirty-year history of the University of Wisconsin's Laboratory for Cancer Research.

Zeit, Walter. "Marquette University School of Medicine: The First Fifty Years." *Wisconsin Medical Journal* 62 (July 1963): 295–302.
The history of a medical school which was formed in 1913 after two Milwaukee proprietary schools received very poor ratings in the Flexner report.

The *Milwaukee Medical Times* published a series of short histories of Milwaukee's hospitals during 1953, 1954, and 1955.

Disease and Public Health

Ackerknecht, Erwin H. "Diseases in the Middle West." In *Essays in the History of Medicine,* edited by the Davis Lecture Committee, pp. 168–81. Chicago: for the Davis Lecture Committee by the University of Illinois Press, 1965.
A historical review of the diseases which affected nineteenth-century Midwest pioneers, including malaria, typhoid fever, dysentery, erysipelas, cholera, smallpox, milk sickness, epidemic meningitis, tuberculosis, and goiter.

Ackerknecht, Erwin H. *Malaria in the Upper Mississippi Valley, 1760–1900.* Baltimore: Johns Hopkins Press, 1945.
A description of the prevalence of malaria in Minnesota, Wisconsin, Iowa, Illinois, and Missouri. Possible factors causing a decrease in malaria cases in these states are discussed; the use of quinine is stressed as a curative, rather than preventive, measure.

Bremer, Gail D. "The Wisconsin Idea and the Public Health Move-
ment, 1890–1915." M.S. thesis, University of Wisconsin, 1963.
A description of the leadership role which some University of Wisconsin faculty took in the public health campaigns to enact industrial hy-
giene legislation, to eradicate tuberculosis, and to provide the public
with pure food and drugs.
Cranefield, Paul F. "Cholera in Wisconsin, 1832–1834." *Wisconsin
Medical Journal* 49 (June 1950): 509–11.
Speculations on how the cholera epidemic spread through the state.
Reasons for the lack of contemporary descriptions of the disease are
also postulated.
Dearholt, Hoyt E. "Glimpses of Pioneer Wisconsin Health Work." *Wis-
consin Medical Journal* 31 (November 1932): 774–78.
A summary of the first report (1876) of the Wisconsin State Board of
Health.
Falk, Victor S. "The Influenza Epidemic of 1918." *Wisconsin Medical
Journal* 75 (August 1976): 31–34.
Reminiscences of several Wisconsin physicians who were either in
practice or in medical school during the epidemic.
"The Good Old Days." *Health in Wisconsin* 22, no. 1 (1976): 12–19.
A brief description of early Wisconsin State Board of Health efforts to
control diphtheria, smallpox, scarlet fever, typhoid fever, and tuber-
culosis.
Harper, Cornelius A. "A Brief Outline of Public Health Development in
Wisconsin." *Wisconsin Medical Journal* 30 (October 1931): 803–6.
A review of the major activities of the Wisconsin State Board of
Health in its first forty years.
Harper, Cornelius A. "History of the Wisconsin State Board of Health."
1949.
A typescript in the State Historical Society of Wisconsin.
Harstad, Peter T. "Disease and Sickness on the Wisconsin Frontier:
Cholera." *Wisconsin Magazine of History* 43 (1959–60): 203–20.
A description of the 1832–1833 and 1849–1853 cholera epidemics in
Wisconsin. The medical profession had few effective remedies, but
Milwaukee officials implemented many preventive measures before
and during the second epidemic.
Harstad, Peter T. "Disease and Sickness on the Wisconsin Frontier:
Smallpox and Other Diseases." *Wisconsin Magazine of History* 43
(1959–60): 253–63.
The effects of smallpox epidemics on both the Indian and white pop-
ulations. Vaccination was a controversial issue, particularly among

Milwaukee's German population. Several other contagious and chronic diseases are briefly described.

Harstad, Peter T. "Health in the Upper Mississippi River Valley, 1820 to 1861." Ph.D. dissertation, University of Wisconsin, 1963.
A study of the factors which influenced the health of Midwest settlers. Geography, climate, housing, and food and water supply were among the environmental factors. Prevalent diseases included malaria, typhoid fever, cholera and tuberculosis. Allopaths as well as sectarians offered various treatments for both epidemic and endemic diseases.

Harstad, Peter T. "Sickness and Disease on the Wisconsin Frontier: Malaria, 1820–1850." *Wisconsin Magazine of History* 43 (1959–60): 83–96.
An account of the devastating effects that endemic and epidemic malaria had on Wisconsin's military forts and civilian settlements. Numerous medical treatments and patent medicines existed; there were also several different explanations of the causation of malaria.

Leavitt, Judith Walzer. "Politics and Public Health: Smallpox in Milwaukee, 1894–95." *Bulletin of the History of Medicine* 50 (Winter 1976): 553–68.
A case example of the relationship between politics and public health. Although many nineteenth-century epidemics helped increase the powers of health departments, this smallpox epidemic resulted in a loss of health department power and in the impeachment of the health commissioner.

Leavitt, Judith Walzer. *The Healthiest City: Milwaukee and the Politics of Health Reform.* Princeton: Princeton University Press, forthcoming.
An examination of the city government's gradually increasing responsibility for the city's public health. Three major areas of Health Department activity are studied in detail: control over infectious disease (smallpox), sanitation (garbage), and food control (milk). Particular emphasis is placed upon the complex relationship between politics and public health.

Leavitt, Judith Walzer. "The Wasteland: Garbage and Sanitary Reform in the Nineteenth Century City." *Journal of the History of Medicine and Allied Sciences* 35 (1980): 431–52.
An exploration of the relationships among politics, economic interests, and sanitary reform from 1875 to 1911 in Milwaukee.

Middleton, William S. "Cholera Epidemics in Iowa County, Wisconsin." *Wisconsin Medical Journal* 37 (October 1938): 894–900.

The impact of the 1849–1851 cholera epidemics on several mining communities in southwestern Wisconsin. Quotations from contemporary letters and newspapers are included.

Wisconsin Historical Records Survey. *A Guide to the Public Vital Statistics Records in Wisconsin.* Madison: Wisconsin Historical Records Survey, 1941.

A documentation of the sources of early vital statistics. Demographic information can be obtained from the decennial United States census, from the State Historical Society collection, and from numerous state publications.

Contributors

Peter T. Harstad, Ph.D., is Director of the State Historical Society of Iowa. He is the author of numerous publications in American history, including a three-part series on "Sickness and Disease on the Wisconsin Frontier" in the *Wisconsin Magazine of History* (1959–60).

Mary Van Hulle Jones, B.S., is a Registered Nurse employed by the University of Wisconsin Extension Department of Nursing. A graduate student in the Department of the History of Science, University of Wisconsin–Madison, she is studying the development of public-health nursing in America.

Elizabeth Barnaby Keeney, M.A., is a doctoral candidate in the Department of the History of Science, University of Wisconsin–Madison. She is writing her dissertation on botany in American culture.

Judith Walzer Leavitt, Ph.D., is Assistant Professor of the History of Medicine, the History of Science, and Women's Studies, University of Wisconsin–Madison. She has coedited *Medicine without Doctors: Home Health Care in American History* (1977) and *Sickness and Health in America: Readings in the History of Medicine and Public Health* (1978), and has written *The Healthiest City: Milwaukee and the Politics of Health Reform* (forthcoming).

Susan Eyrich Lederer, M.A., is a doctoral candidate in the history of science and medicine at the University of Wisconsin–Madison. She is completing a dissertation on the history of animal and human experimentation in America.

Edmond P. Minihan, M.A., is Special Assistant to the Administrator, Division of Health, Department of Health and Social Services, State of Wisconsin. As a graduate student in medical sociology at the University of Wisconsin–Madison, he studied the development of sectarian medicine. He is author of articles in *Administrative Science Quarterly* and *Hospitals*.

Ronald L. Numbers, Ph.D., is Professor of the History of Medicine and the History of Science and Chairman of the Department of the History of Medicine, University of Wisconsin–Madison. He has written or edited a number of books, including, most recently, *The Education of American Physicians: Historical Essays* (1980).

Guenter B. Risse, M.D., Ph.D., is Professor of the History of Medicine and the History of Science, University of Wisconsin–Madison. In addition to writing numerous articles in the history of medicine, he has edited *Modern China and Traditional Chinese Medicine* (1973), has coedited *Medicine without Doctors: Home Health Care in American History* (1977), and has translated K. E. Rothschuh's *History of Physiology* (1973).

Philip Shoemaker, M.A., is a doctoral candidate in the Department of the History of Science, University of Wisconsin–Madison, where he is writing a dissertation on Ormsby McKnight Mitchel and the development of astronomy in nineteenth-century America. He is the author of an article on spiritualism in nineteenth-century Wisconsin (*Journal of Religious Studies*, 1979).

Deanna Reed Springall, M.A., is Data Manager/Evaluation Specialist, East Alabama Emergency Medical Services, Anniston, Alabama. As a graduate student in the history of medicine at the University of Wisconsin–Madison, she studied the history of public health in America.

Dale E. Treleven, M.A., is a fifth-generation descendant of a pioneer Wisconsin family. Before joining the staff of the State Historical Society of Wisconsin as research historian and director of the state oral history program, he spent three years as research coordinator with the Department of Family Medicine and Practice, University of Wisconsin–Madison. His primary research interests are in agricultural and rural history.

Index

Accidents: burns, 55; farm, 146; fractures and dislocations, 28; hernias, 28; mentioned, 26, 108
A. C. Club of Milwaukee, 87–88
Ackerknecht, Erwin H., 184
Allopaths. *See* Regulars
American College of Surgeons, 120
American Dispensatory, 135
American Indians: Chippewa, 4, 5; diseases of, 5; Fox, 4; Kickapoo, 4; Mascouten, 4; Menominee, 4; Miami, 4; Ottawa, 4; Potawatomi, 4, 5; religion and medicine, 5; Sauk, 4; therapies, 5; Winnebago, 4, 5, 6
American Medical Association: Council on Medical Education, 182; House of Delegates, 90; survey of regular medical societies, 88; survey of United States physicians, 49; mentioned, 37, 85, 91, 95, 97n9, 124, 144
American Public Health Association, 8, 172
Anesthesia, 8, 108, 121
Animal Magnetism, 17
Antisepsis. *See* Asepsis
Appleton, Wis., 77, 135, 137
Arries, Mrs. Crecentia, 60, 61
Asepsis: Lister, 30; and surgery, 30, 33, 37, 78, 108–10, 121; mentioned, 8, 108
Asheville, North Carolina, 115
Ashland, Wis., 35, 111, 112
Associated Women of the American Farm Bureau Federation, 144
Association of American Medical Colleges, 180, 182
Association of Medical Superintendents of American Institutions for the Insane, 82
Aurora, Wis., 139

Babcock, Wis., 83
Baraboo, Wis., 53

Bardeen, Charles R., 34, 37, 38, 114, 142, 150n51, 178, 183, 184
Barron County, Wis., 146
Bartlett, Edwin, 81
Bartlett, J. K., 84
Bascom, John, 84, 178
Bascom Hall, 178
Battle Creek, Michigan, 56
Battle Creek Sanitarium, Battle Creek, Michigan, 56, 57
Bayfield County, Wis., 138
Beach, Dr. Wooster, 53
Beaumont, William, 3, 14, 106
Becker, Captain, hospital patient, 110
Beebe, Loran, 32
Beloit, Wis., 49
Berlin, Wis., 30, 54
Biemiller, Andrew J., 95
Birge, Edward A., 178
Blackburn, Dr. A. T., 29
Black Hawk War of 1832, 16
Blue Mound Sanatorium, 116
Blue Shield plan, 95
Bonner, Thomas N., 4
Boscobel, Wis., 145
Bossard, Dr. Marcus, 34
Botanical doctors (steam doctors), 26
Bowen, James, 51
Brett, B. C., 92
Brickbauer, Dr. George, 52
Brittingham, T. E., 120
Brown County Medical Society, 90
Buley, R. Carlyle, 4
Burlington, Iowa, 14
Burnham's Canal, 161

Camp Randall, Madison, Wis., 41
Carnegie Foundation, 183
Carroll College, 180, 181

Carver, Jonathan, 5
Castleman, Dr. Alfred L., 82, 84, 111–12
Catholic, 106, 108, 111, 120
Chapman, Chandler B., 179
Cherry, Essie, 62
Cherry, Leslie, 62
Chesbrough, Ellis Sylvester, 160
Chicago, Illinois, 30, 49, 53, 160, 177, 178
Chicago Board of Health, 62
Chippewa County, Wis., 138
Chippewa Falls, Wis., 30
Chiropractic: definition, 65; legal confu-
    sion with osteopathy, 66–67; "mixers" vs.
    "straights," 68; public attitudes toward,
    69; public confusion with osteopathy, 65–
    66; rural appeal, 59, 68; societies, 67,
    68–69; mentioned, 59, 65–69. See also
    Chiropractors
Chiropractors: fees, 59; legal right to prac-
    tice, 67; legal use of "doctor," 69; number
    in Illinois, 65; number in Iowa, 65, 68;
    number in Minnesota, 65; number in
    United States, 65; number in Wisconsin,
    65, 68; separate state examining board,
    67; women, 59; mentioned, 47, 59, 65–
    69. See also Chiropractic
Christensen, Christian, 36–37
Christian Science: definition, 60; "dispen-
    saries" (reading rooms), 60; fees of heal-
    ers, 61; number of healers in Illinois, 65;
    number of healers in Iowa, 65; number
    of healers in Minnesota, 65; number of
    healers in United States, 65; number of
    healers in Wisconsin, 65, 68; prosecution
    of healers, 60; state licensing, 59; urban
    appeal, 73n66; women healers, 59, 72n61;
    mentioned, 47, 59–61
Cleveland Homeopathic Hospital College,
    49
Colfax, Wis., 138
College of Physicians and Surgeons, Kan-
    sas City, Missouri, 61
Coney, William H., 180
Coney Medical Institute. See Milwaukee
    College of Physicians and Surgeons
Contagion-anticontagion controversy, 90
Cooper, James, 135
Crane, Horace O., 27–28
Croghan, General George, 105
Crownhart, Charles, 96

Crownhart, George, 96
Cumberland, Wis., 69

Dane County, Wis., 88
Dane County Medical Society, 90
Darling, Dr. M. C., 76
Davenport, Iowa, 66, 179
Davis, Warren B., 62
Dayton, Wis., 139
Death rates: among children, 156, 164; and
    housing density, 158; decreasing at end of
    nineteenth century, 166; from cancer,
    145; from diphtheria, 32, 140; from dys-
    entery, diarrhea, and enteritis, 140; from
    influenza, 146–47; from malaria, 7; from
    meningitis, 140; from pneumonia, 140,
    146–47; from tuberculosis, 117, 128n54;
    135; from typhoid fever, 140; from
    whooping cough, 140; hospital, 108; in
    Milwaukee, 168; in Wisconsin, 168; in-
    fant, 140, 165, 166, 170, 174n39; mater-
    nal, 140; rural vs. urban, 140, 169, 170;
    surgical patients, 108; urban, 156
Dentistry: fees, 28; licensing, 87; num-
    ber in Wisconsin, 145; mentioned, 17, 20,
    100n69
Desmoine County, Wisconsin Territory, 13
Diagnostic techniques: auscultation, 27;
    clinical thermometer, 27; Kolmer syphi-
    lis test, 37; laryngoscope, 30; lumbar
    puncture, 32; microscope, 31; ophthal-
    moscope, 30; percussion, 27; pulse, 27;
    serological tests, 37; sphygmomanome-
    ter, 32; stethoscope, 30; tongue charac-
    teristics, 27; Wassermann test, 36; Widal
    agglutination reaction, 33; x-rays, 33, 37,
    120
Diamond Bluff, Wis., 62
Diseases: ague, 7, 14; alcoholism, 108; an-
    gina pectoris, 31; appendicitis, 121; arth-
    ritis, 146; Bright's disease, 110; burns, 55;
    cancer, 145; catarrh, 106; chilblains, 29;
    cholera, 7, 15, 16, 26, 35, 49, 90, 106;
    cholera infantum, 157; debility, 108; dia-
    betes, 37; diphtheria, 7, 26, 31–32, 35,
    134, 135, 137, 139, 140, 156, 158, 159,
    163, 166, 167; dropsy, 5; dysentery, 7, 8,
    26, 106, 140, 157, 159; enteritis, 140; epi-
    lepsy, 142; erysipelas, 7, 108; faced by
    pioneers, 7; goiter, 142; heart disease,

145, 146; hysteria, 108; influenza, 5, 114, 121, 146–47; insanity, 108, 150n51; intermittent fever, 106, 108; malaria, 7, 8, 14, 19, 26, 106, 108; measles, 5, 7, 135; meningitis, 32, 61, 140; mental, 138; mumps, 135; nervousness, 108; ophthalmia, 106; otitis, 36; paralysis, 5, 108; pleurisy, 108; pneumonia, 26, 108, 114, 135, 140, 147, 158; puerperal eclampsia, 31; puerperal fever, 78; rheumatic fever, 36; rheumatism, 55, 106, 108; rural, 134–35; scarlatina, 55, 163; scarlet fever, 7, 134, 135, 158, 165; smallpox, 5, 7, 26, 29, 31, 35, 106, 134, 166; stroke, 31; "summer complaint," 157; tuberculosis, 8, 26, 31, 32, 35, 36, 79, 108, 114, 115–18, 128n54, 135, 157, 171; tumors, 108; typhoid fever, 7, 8, 26, 29, 31, 33, 35, 108, 134, 135, 137, 139, 140, 158, 159, 163; typhus, 134; venereal, 5, 36, 37; whooping cough, 55, 140; yellow fever, 35
Dix, Dorothea, 111
Dr. Ravn's Hospital, 113
Dodd, J. M., 35
Dodge, Dr. E. F., 30
Dodge, Henry, 13, 16
Dodge County, Wis., 28, 137, 139
Door County, Wis., 50
Douglas, James S., 48–49, 51
Douglas County, Wis., 95
Downer College, 109
Drake, Daniel: etiology of malaria, 14–15
Dubuque County, Wis., 13
Duffy, John, 4
Dunn County, Wis., 135

Eau Claire, Wis., 49, 53, 111, 125
Eclectics: cooperation with allopaths, 86; decline, 58; definition, 53; distribution in United States, 53; distribution in Wisconsin, 53; medical school, 53; medical society, 53; percent of Wisconsin physicians, 53, 92; mentioned, 47, 53–54, 58, 65, 75, 84, 86, 92, 148n22
Eddy, Mary Baker, 59–60
Edwards, Dr. Tom O., 41n11
Ehrlich, Paul, 37
Elba, Wis., 139
Elkhart Lake, Wis., 52
Ellington, Wis., 135

Elliott, Dr. Thomas, 113
Elmergreen, Ralph, 60–61, 64
England, 123
Epidemics: cholera, 26, 49, 90; influenza, 121, 146–47; smallpox, 5, 106, 135, 139; mentioned, 138
Epley, F. W., 34
Erie Canal, 6
Erlanger, Joseph, 178
Ethnic groups: Cornish, 133; English, 21; German, 49, 108, 114, 137, 158, 173n13; Irish, 108, 114, 137; Norwegian, 138; Polish, 137, 158; Scotch, 21; Yankee, 21
Evergreen Park Cottage Sanatorium, 116

Farr, Coryden S., 97n4
Favill, Dr. John, 30, 81
Favill, H. B., 34
Fitchburg, Wis., 28
Flexner, Abraham, 182, 183
Flexner Report of 1910, 37, 142, 182, 183
Fond du Lac, Wis., 30, 49, 77, 78, 81, 133, 155
Fond du Lac Medical Society, 88
Ford, Dr. Julia, 49
Ford, Richard I., 5
Fort Atkinson, Wis., 58
Fort Crawford, Wis., 7, 14, 105, 106
Fort Howard, Wis., 14, 15, 105, 106
Fort Mackinac, Michigan, 106
Fort Winnebago, Wis., 14, 15, 105, 106
Fountain, Wis., 159
Fox, Dr. William (of Milwaukee), 87
Fox, William H., 28
Fox River, 15
Fox River Valley, 91, 106
Frank, Dr. Louis F., 90

Galena, Wis., 15
Galesville University, 179
Genesee, Wis., 19
Germany, 32, 37
Germ theory of disease, 31, 79
Glasgow Royal Infirmary, 18
Graham, Dr. David, 50
Grayson, Robert L., 68
Green Bay, Wis., 6, 14, 28, 105, 155, 159
Gridley Dairy, Milwaukee, Wis., 165
Griffith, Dr. William, 22
Ground, William C., 33

Guide for Women, 135
Gundersen, Dr. Adolf, 36–37, 110

Hahnemann, Samuel, 48, 135
Hahnemann Medical College, Chicago, Illinois, 49
Hahnemann Medical College, St. Louis, Missouri, 56
Hale, Wis., 139
Hall, Dr. W. W., 138
Harper, Cornelius A., 41, 150
Hayes, Mrs. Mary, 118
Hayes Hospital, 118
Hayward, Wis., 141
Health insurance: Blue Cross, 124, 125; contract medicine, 18; group insurance, 124–25; Marinette and Menominee Hospital Company, 30; Medicaid, 125, 131n109; Medicare, 125, 131n109; Peshtigo Company, 29–30; St. Joseph Hospital, 112; "ticket hospitals," 111, 113; mentioned, 94–96, 103n114
Health statutes: against fee splitting, 36; Eugenics Law of 1913, 35–36; Harrison Narcotic Act of 1914 (U.S.), 36; Hospital Survey and Construction Act (U.S.), 125, 131n109, 144; legalized dissection, 79; Local Health Boards (1883), 139; Marine Hospital Service Act of 1798 (U.S.), 107; Occupational Diseases Act of 1911, 35; Wisconsin territory, 16
Henni, John Martin, 106
Hess, John, 79
Hippocrates, 25
History of Medicine in Louisiana, 4
Hobbins, Joseph, 41n7
Homeopathic Medical Reporter, 48
Homeopathic Medical Society of the State of Wisconsin: licensing laws, 86; membership, 51, 56, 86; mentioned, 51, 56, 58, 102–3n109
Homeopaths: conflicts with allopaths, 48; cooperation with allopaths, 86; distribution in Wisconsin, 49; education, 49–50; medical research, 51–53; percent of Illinois physicians, 70n12; percent of Iowa physicians, 70n12; percent of Michigan physicians, 70n12; percent of Minnesota physicians, 70n12; percent of Rhode Island physicians, 70n12; percent of Wisconsin physicians, 49, 92; pharmacies, 48; women, 49; mentioned, 17, 26, 47, 48–53, 58, 65, 75, 84, 86, 92, 148n22. *See also* Homeopathy
Homeopathy: decline, 58; definition, 48; do-it-yourself guides and kits, 50–51; ethnic tendencies, 49; Medical Society, 48, 86; water cures, 55; mentioned, 48–53, 58, 60, 81. *See also* Homeopaths
Hospital insurance. *See* Health insurance
Hospitals: aseptic surgery, 30, 33, 37, 78, 108–10, 121; dramatic growth in numbers, 37; financial problems, 124; Hill-Burton Program, 125, 131n109, 144; Hospital Survey and Construction Act (U.S.), 125, 131n109, 144; Indians, 141; insane asylums, 82, 111–14, 141–42, 150n51, 169; laboratory medicine, 37; maternity, 120; medical practice shift to, 34; Milwaukee pesthouse, 106, 107; number in United States, 105; number in Wisconsin, 115, 118; number of church-related, 118; number of tuberculosis hospitals in Wisconsin, 117; nursing schools, 123; physician interns, 123–24; population-hospital bed ratios, 125, 169; relation to Catholic Sisters, 111; rise of, 8; rural, 141–42, 143, 144–45; "sick poor," 169; smallpox, 109; "ticket hospital," 111; Toner survey, 110–11; tuberculosis sanitoria, 115–18, 169; United States Army, 105–6; veterans, 141; mentioned, 105–25, 169
Houghton, Dr. Douglass, 5
Hustisford, Wis., 137
Hydropaths: fees, 55; water cures, 54–57; mentioned, 17, 26, 47, 54–57, 75. *See also* Hydropathy
Hydropathy: definition, 54; treatments, 55; mentioned, 6, 54–57. *See also* Hydropaths
Hydrotherapy. *See* Hydropathy

Illinois, 7, 53, 64, 65, 86, 91, 178, 179, 183, 184
Immigrants: source of disease, 106; source of insanity, 82
Indian Doctor's Indian Receipt Book, 135
Indiana, 7, 53, 113
Infinitesimal doses, 48
International Harvest Company, 94

Iowa, 7, 13, 62, 64, 65, 68, 86, 91, 178, 179, 183, 184
Irregulars. *See* Sectarians

Jackson, Arnold S., 37
Jackson, Dr. Reginald, 120
Jackson, Sr., James H., 37
Jackson Clinic, Madison, Wis., 37
Janesville, Wis., 32, 49, 54, 62, 76, 77
Janssen, Jacob S.: first use of x-ray in Wisconsin, 33
Jefferson County, Wis., 27
Jermain, Louis J., 182, 183
Johns Hopkins University, 178, 184
Johnson, G. W., 66
Journal of the American Medical Association, 65
Joys Brothers Co., 32

Kansas, 99n61
Kansas Doctor, 4
Kellogg, Dr. John Harvey, 56, 57
Kenosha, Wis., 49, 54, 68, 155, 167
Kentucky, 91
Keokuk, Iowa, 179
Keshena, Wis., 141
Kilbourn City, Wis., 54
Kirksville, Missouri, 62
Kneipp, Sebastian, 55
Koch, Robert, 79
Koehler, Glenn, 69
Kolb, John, 143
Kurtz, Chester, 40

La Crosse, Wis., 9, 36, 53, 56, 66, 67, 110, 125, 155, 165, 167, 179, 180
La Crosse County Medical Society, 179
La Crosse Medical College, 179-80
Lafayette County, Wis., 135, 139
Lake Muskego, Wis., 7
Lake Nebagamon, Wis., 116
Lake-Side Retreat, 55
Lake Side Water-Cure, 54, 55
Lancaster, Wis., 145
Landis, Dr. S. M., 55
Langlade County Medical Society, 80
Lapham, Increase, 7
Law of similars, 48
Life expectancy: general population, 3; increased, 41

Linning, Charles, 67
Little Lake Tomahawk, Wis., 116, 118
London, England, 17, 19, 20
Lone Rock, Wis., 146
Lumbering, 29, 111, 113

McCormack, Dr. J. N., 91
MacCornack, R. L., 146
McWilliams, Dr., fictional physician, 40
Madison, Wis.: board of health, 159; mentioned, 6, 9, 15, 30, 37, 40, 41n7, 49, 53, 54, 55, 56, 67, 73n66, 76, 77, 82, 88, 90, 100n69, 111, 113, 118, 125, 136, 155, 177, 178, 179, 180, 183, 184
Madison General Hospital: contagious disease, 121; group insurance, 125; number of beds, 118, 120; number of cases, 122, 124; nursing school, 123; out-patient care, 121; patient costs, 121, 123, 124; staff size, 120-21; surgery, 121; mentioned, 118-25
Madison General Hospital Association, 118, 124
Madison Medical College, 179
Madison Sanitarium, 56, 57, 120
Madison Water-Cure, 55, 56
Mall, Franklin P., 178
Manitowoc County, Wis., 110
Manual of Homeopathic Practice, 50
Marine Hospital, 107
Marinette, Wis., 29, 111
Marquette University School of Medicine, 181-83
Marshfield, Wis., 9, 36, 125
Marshfield Clinic, 36, 144
Martin, Dr. S. J., 50
Maryland, 99n61, 106
Massachusetts Metaphysical College, 60
Mayo Clinic, Rochester, Minnesota, 152n81
Mayville, Wis., 139
Mazomanie, Wis., 28
Meachem, Jr., James G., 31
Medical College of Wisconsin, 183, 184
Medical Defense plan, 35
Medical journals, 75
Medical Reserve Corps, 36
Medical Schools in Wisconsin, 62-63, 177-84
Medical societies: "black list," 88; discipline of ethics, 90; fee bills, 88, 89, 93; health

Continued:
insurance interest, 94–96; legal permission to incorporate, 75–76; local, 87–91; regular open membership to sectarians, 92; regular prohibit member contact with sectarians, 48, 90; mentioned, 75–96
Medical Society of the Territory of Wisconsin, 76. *See also* Wisconsin State Medical Society
Mendota, Lake, 113
Mendota State Hospital for the Insane: patient profile, 114; recovery rate, 114; staff, 113; mentioned, 22, 82, 111, 113–14, 118
Menomonee Marsh, 161
Menomonee River, 161
Mental illness: hospitals, 82; rural, 138; Wisconsin State Medical Society concern, 82
Merrill, Wis., 111, 113
Methodist, 61
Michigan, 7, 106, 178, 183, 184
Michigan, Lake, 6, 15, 80, 155, 160, 163
Michigan Territory, 16
Middleton, William S., 183
Middleton Depot, Wis., 28
The Midwest Pioneer: His Ills, Cures & Doctors, 4
Midwifery, 100n69, 101n77, 142
Miller, Simon, 42n16
Miller, William Snow, 178, 184
Milwaukee, Wis.: antivaccination group, 166; cremation plant, 164; death in city, 157–58; ethnic profile, 108, 158; garbage, 157, 162, 163–64; "healthiest" large city, 172; housing problems, 156–57; mortality rates, 168; population, 8, 106; urban cow barns, 164–65; water supplies, 160–61; mentioned, 6, 8, 15, 21, 29, 30, 32, 34, 35, 48, 49, 51, 53, 60, 61, 62, 68, 73n66, 76, 77, 78, 81, 82, 86, 87, 88, 94, 95, 106, 109, 111, 116, 118, 119, 125, 134, 135, 155–72, 177, 178, 180, 181, 182, 183
Milwaukee Academy of Medicine, 51, 87
Milwaukee Board of Health. *See* Milwaukee Department of Health
Milwaukee City Medical Association, 48, 90, 108
Milwaukee College of Physicians and Surgeons, 180

Milwaukee County, Wis., 40, 91, 95
Milwaukee County Hospital, 111
Milwaukee County Medical Society: health insurance, 103n120; mentioned, 20, 94
Milwaukee Department of Health, 32, 160, 161, 162, 163, 164, 166, 167
Milwaukee Health Center, 94
Milwaukee Institute (College) of Osteopathy, 62, 63, 180
Milwaukee Medical College and School of Dentistry, 182
Milwaukee Medical Journal, 61, 64
Milwaukee Medical Society, 81, 88
Milwaukee River, 161
Milwaukee Sentinel, 87
Milwaukee University, 180
Mineral Point, Wis., 6, 13, 76, 77
Minneapolis, Minnesota, 62
Minnesota, 13, 37, 64, 65, 66, 86, 91, 178, 183, 184
Missionary Nurses' Training School, 56
Mississippi River, 6, 13, 14, 15, 62, 105
Missouri, 7, 53, 62, 64, 65
Mitchell, John, 26
Mondovi, Wis., 42n16
Monona, Lake, 55, 56
Monopoly, 16, 86
Morikubo, Shegataro, 66–67
Morris and Hartwell (La Crosse, Wis., law firm), 67
Mortality rates. *See* Death rates
Mt. Horeb, Wis., 28
Mueller, Armin, 35
Mukwonago, Wis., 17, 22

Naples, Wis., 159
National Health Honor Roll, 172
Native Americans. *See* American Indians
Naturopathy, 59
Neopit, Wis., 141
New Guide to Health, 135
New Jersey, 99n61
New Richmond, Wis., 135, 137
New York, 48, 53, 55, 110, 114, 166
New York City, New York, 55, 156
New York City Board of Health, 8
New York State Medical Society, 76
Nichols, Miss Emma, 60, 61
Nightingale, Florence, 123
North Dakota, 13

Northern Institute of Osteopathy, Minneapolis, Minnesota, 62
Northern State Hospital for the Insane: patient profile, 114; mentioned, 111, 114
Norway, 110
Nursing: public health, 141, 142; schools, 56, 123

Obstetrics: home vs. hospital deliveries, 121; mentioned, 53, 108
Oconto, Wis., 59
Ohio, 50, 53
Omro, Wis., 133
Oneida County, Wis., 116
Oregon, Wis., 28
Organon of Homeopathic Medicine, 135
Orthodox physicians. *See* Regulars
Osceola, Wis., 145
Oshkosh, Wis., 49, 79, 90, 111, 114, 155
Osler, William, 33
Osteopaths: education, 62; fees, 59, 62; inclusion in Wisconsin State Medical Society, 65; legal right to perform surgery, 65; number in Illinois, 64–65; number in Iowa, 64–65; number in Minnesota, 64–65; number in United States, 65; number in Wisconsin, 64–65, 68, 73n81, 92; prosecution, 62–64; state licensing, 59, 64, 86; women, 59; mentioned, 47, 59, 61–65, 67. *See also* Osteopathy
Osteopathy: definition, 61; "mixers" vs. "purists," 65; rural appeal, 59; schools, 62; mentioned, 59, 61–65, 66, 67. *See also* Osteopaths
Outagamie County, Wis., 135
Owen, Robert, 17
Ozaukee County, Wis., 135

Painesville, Ohio, 50
Palmer, B. J., 67
Palmer, Daniel David, 65, 66, 67, 68
Palmer College of Chiropractic, Davenport, Iowa, 67
Palmer Institute and Chiropractic Infirmary, Davenport, Iowa, 66
Palmyra, Wis., 54
Paoli, Wis., 28
Paris, France, 17
Passavant Hospital, 111
Patent medicine: attraction to rural citizens, 135–37, 146; mentioned, frontispiece, 83, 87, 146
Peck, George W. (Governor), 33
Pennsylvania State Medical Society, 103n115
Peshtigo Company, 29
Peshtigo Harbor Lumber Camp, 29
Pharmacists (druggists), 33, 98n41
Philadelphia, Pennsylvania, 55
Phreno-magnetism, 17
Physicians: apprenticeship, 26, 27, 50, 177, 183; competition, 35, 84; decline of rural practice, 40, 68, 142–43, 145; earnings, 20, 28, 40; education, 177–84; fees, 27, 28, 29, 30, 89, 93; form of patient payment, 18, 29; group practice, 36–37, 45n88, 144; hospital interns, 123–24, 131n93; malpractice regulation, 35; malpractice suits, 28, 34–35, 81; number in Wisconsin, 140–41, 170; office use, 33; personal health, 36; practice of regular, 17–22; public advertising, 81; public distrust, 35, 36; specialization, 34, 40, 142; status, 26, 18, 20, 28, 38–40, 137; urban, 170. *See also* Regulars; Restrictive legislation; Sectarians; entries for individual sects
Physicians Alliance, 96
Physicians Business Association of Sheboygan, 93
Pickard, Madge E., 4
Pinkham, Lydia, 135
Polk's Medical and Surgical Register, 111
Portage, Wisconsin, 6, 14, 105
Port Washington, Wis., 135
Poudrette doctors, 17
Practical Homeopathy for the People, 51
Prairie du Chien, Wis., 6, 7, 14, 105
Prairie du Sac, Wis., 97n4
Prepaid medical care. *See* Health insurance
Priessnitz, Vincenz, 54
Public health: food quality, 164–65, 168; fresh-air schools, 171; full-time officers, 167; garbage, 163–64, 168; inoculation efforts, 142; laws, 61; local health boards, 139–40, 159, 166; local medical society support, 90; nursing, 141, 142; pressures against, 168–69; privy vaults, 161–63, 168; rural health, 133–47, 159; rural sanitation, 138–39; rural vs. urban, 169; sewer gas, 163; state board of

Continued:
  health, 138, 140; vaccination efforts, 166; water supplies, 160–61, 168; mentioned, 81–84, 138–47, 155–72
— Wisconsin State Medical Society support: abortion, 82–83; homes for unwed mothers, 83; obscenity, 82–84; mentioned, 81–84

Quackery, 17, 26, 65, 87, 146. *See also* Quacks
Quacks, 26, 47, 56, 58, 64, 85, 86, 100n69, 137. *See also* Quackery

Racine, Wis., frontispiece, 50, 62, 77, 111, 155
Racine County, Wis., 135
Racine Medical Association, 88
Redelings, T. J., 94
Reed, Dr. Thomas, 114
Reeve, Dr. J. T., 77, 86
Reeve, John C., 28
Regulars: percent of Wisconsin physicians, 53, 92; mentioned, 21, 25–41, 47, 49, 51, 53, 56, 58, 60, 61, 64, 68, 75, 84, 85, 86, 137, 148n22, 178, 180
Restrictive legislation: basic science act, 68; chiropractors free to practice, 67; state board of dental examiners, 87; mentioned, 100n69
— State board of medical examiners: osteopaths included, 64, 86; mentioned, 58, 59, 64, 86
Richland County, Wis., 139, 146
Riddell, Dr. S. S., 30
River Pines Sanatorium, 116
Rocci, Riva, 32
Rock County, Wis., 95
Rock Island Medical College, Illinois, 179
Rock River Medical Society, 88
Roentgen, Wilhelm, 33
Ross, Dr., Painesville, Ohio, physician, 50
Ross, Dr. Laura J., 81
Rowley, Newman C., 28
Rush Medical College, 62

St. Croix County, Wis., 135, 146
St. Francis Hospital, 110
St. John's Infirmary. *See* St. Mary's Hospital, Milwaukee, Wis.

St. Joseph Hospital, 112
St. Louis, Missouri, 56
St. Luke's Hospital, 111
St. Martin, Alexis, 106
St. Mary's Eye and Ear Infirmary, Milwaukee, Wis., 51
St. Mary's Hospital, Madison, Wis., 120
St. Mary's Hospital, Milwaukee, Wis.: finances, 107, 110; Marine Hospital, 107; mortality rate, 108; nursing school, 123; patient fees, 110; patient profile, 108; physician support, 107; surgical patient mortality rate, 108; mentioned, 8, 106–10, 118, 119
Sauk City, Wis., 28
Sauk County Medical Society, 82
Sawyer, Jenny, 60
Sawyer, Silas, 60
Schue, Dr. Alexander, 90
Science and Health, 60
Sectarians: percent of Wisconsin physicians, 47; mentioned, 47–69, 85, 86, 90, 92, 137, 178, 180. *See also* Physicians; entries for individual sects
Senn, Nicholas, 30, 78–79, 86
Seventh-day Adventist, 56, 120
Shawano, Wis., 144
Sheboygan, Wis., 35, 54, 73n66, 155, 159
Sheldon, Dr. C. S., 77, 79–80, 84, 91, 92
Sherman, Lewis, 51
Sherman Anti-Trust Act, 95
Shullsburg, Wis., 139
Sisters of Charity, 106, 107
Smith, Dr. W. H., 124
Society of Equality (Equalitarians), 17, 18, 19
Society of Wisconsin Chiropractors (SWC): "mixers," 68; mentioned, 68–69
South Dakota, 13
Spring, Lake, 17
Spring Green, Wis., 29, 34
State Medical Society of Wisconsin. *See* Wisconsin State Medical Society
Statistical Report on the Sickness and Mortality in the Army of the United States (1840), 14
Steel, Dr. Thomas, 17–22
Stevens, Dr. J. V., 28
Stevens Point, Wis., 116
Still, Andrew Taylor, 61, 65

Still, Charles, 62
Stoughton, Wis., 28
Superior, Wis., 32, 33, 155
Surgeons: fees, 27; number in Wisconsin, 140–41. *See also* Surgery
Surgery: anesthesia, 8, 108, 121; appendectomies, 34, 110, 121; aseptic, 30, 33, 37, 78, 108–10, 121; carbolic acid, 30; changing practice, 30; chloroform, 27; hospitals, 108, 110, 121; hysterectomies, 34; intubation, 32; kitchen surgery, 110; ovariotomies, 34; tracheotomy, 32; mentioned, 16, 53, 56, 108. *See also* Surgeons

Telephone, 8, 34, 140
Therapeutics and Materia Medica for the Use of Families and Physicians, 51
Therapies: abortion, 82–83, 183; allopathic, 49; antimeningococcic serum, 32; antiphlogistic, 26; antipyrine. *See* salicylic acid; arsphenamine, 37; blood letting, 17, 27, 31, 47, 48, 75; blistering, 17; botanics. *See* herbal; calomel, 27; cataplasms, 17; chloral hydrate, 31; coagulants, 5; diet, 56; diphtheria antitoxin, 32, 166; Dover powder, 27; electrotherapy, 56; emetics, 5; epsom salts, 27, 29; febrifuges, 5; herbal, 5, 53, 75, 135; "heroic," 27, 47; homeopathic, 135; home remedies, 135; hydrotherapy, 6, 54–57, 120; injections, 17; inoculation, 142; insulin, 37; iodine pills, 142; ipecac, 27; jalap, 27; lancets, 19, 27, 53; laudanum, 27; laxatives, 5; leeching, 17; massotherapy, 56; moral therapy, 111, 113; morphine, 19; nitroglycerine, 31; opium, 27; poultices, 17; purging, 17, 27, 47, 75; quinine, 19, 20, 27, 29; salicylic acid, 31; serotherapy, 32; smallpox vaccine, 19, 166; stimulating, 26; streptomycin, 117; tartar emetic, 27; tetanus antitoxin, 32; tranquilizers, 114; vaccination, 158; vomiting, 17, 27; x-ray, 33, 120
Thompson, Swen A. L., 62, 64
Thomson, Samuel, 135
Till, John, 146
Toftness, L. S., 69
Tokyo Academy of Science, Tokyo, Japan, 67
Tomah, Wis., 141

Toner, J. M., 110
Trall, Dr. Russell T., 55
Transactions of the Wisconsin State Medical Society, 31
Transportation: ambulance, 109, 142; automobile, 8, 38–40; carriage, 20, 28; cutter, 28; foot, 18, 28; horseback, 20, 28; sleigh, 20, 28; mentioned, 137, 140
Treatise . . . on the Principal Diseases of the Interior Valley of North America (1850), 15
Trempealeau County, Wis., 137, 139, 146, 179
Trevitt, Dr. A. W., 111
Turtle Lake, Wis., 146

United States Army, 14, 105
United States Commissioner of Agriculture, 138
University of Glasgow, Scotland, 17
University of London, England, 17
University of Wisconsin: College of Engineering, 69; four-year Medical School, 183, 184; history of medicine, 183–84; Medical School "on paper," 177–78; premedical course, 178; School of Agriculture, 115; Student Health Service, 183; two-year Medical School, 177–78, 183; mentioned, 84, 120, 142, 143, 180
University of Wisconsin Medical School. *See* University of Wisconsin
Urine doctors, 17

Van Dusen, Dr. Harmon, 76, 77, 81
Veterinarians, 100n69

Wabasha, Wis., 66
Walbridge, Dr. J. S., 30
Waldo, Wis., 29
Wales, Wis., 116, 117, 128
Washburn, Dr. William H., 25
Water-Cure Journal, 55
Water Cures: homeopathic, 55; hydropathic, 54–57
Waterford, Wis., 135
Watertown, Wis., 32
Waukesha (Prairieville), Wis., 20, 33
Waukesha County, Wis., 19, 21, 89, 116
Waupaca County, Wis., 141
Waupaca County Medical Society, 88

Wausau, Wis., 53, 111
Waushara County, Wis., 139
Wauwatosa, Wis., 107
Western Medical Society of Wisconsin, 28
Weston, Dr., Madison, Wis., physician, 15
Whipple, E. J., 66
White, Ellen G., 56
Whitehall Clinic, 146
Whiting, J. B., 84
Whyte, Dr. William, 32
Willard, Dr. Horace B., 27
Winnebago, Lake, 144
Winnebago County Medical Society, 79, 88
Wisconsin Anti-Tuberculosis Association,
    171
Wisconsin Central Medical Association,
    88, 90
Wisconsin Chiropractic Association (WCA):
    "straights," 68; mentioned, 67, 68–69
Wisconsin College of Physicians and Sur-
    geons, 180–83
Wisconsin Eclectic Medical College, 53,
    180
Wisconsin General Hospital, 183
Wisconsin Hospital Association, 123, 124
Wisconsin Hospital Construction Plan, 144
Wisconsin Medical College, 180
Wisconsin Medical Journal, 34, 39, 83
Wisconsin Medical Union of Physicians and
    Surgeons, 100–101n74

Wisconsin Osteopath, 59
Wisconsin Physicians Service, 95, 103n120
Wisconsin Plan, 95
Wisconsin River, 15
Wisconsin State Dental Society, 87
Wisconsin State Eclectic Medical Society:
    licensing laws, 86; mentioned, 53
Wisconsin State Medical Society: blocks
    University of Wisconsin Medical School,
    178; discipline of ethics, 81; health edu-
    cation and hygiene, 84–85; health insur-
    ance, 94–96; Hospital for the Insane, 82;
    joins AMA, 91; legislative efforts, 79, 82;
    licensing laws, 85–87; malpractice suits,
    81; membership, 77, 81, 91; mentally ill,
    82; public health, 81–84; purpose, 77;
    regulars, 77; relations with irregulars,
    85–87; reorganized, 77; scientific medi-
    cine, 78–79; social events, 79–81; stand-
    ing committees, 78; supports pre-medical
    course at University of Wisconsin, 84;
    supports tuberculosis sanatoria, 99n45;
    mentioned, 35, 64, 76–87, 91, 92, 94, 96,
    97n9
Wood County, Wis., 144
Wright, Gilbert, 21

Youmans, Dr. Henry A., 21–22
Youmans, Dr. Jeremiah, 22
Young, William M., 179

JACKET DESIGNED BY CAROLINE BECKETT
COMPOSED BY METRICOMP, GRUNDY CENTER, IOWA
MANUFACTURED BY NORTH CENTRAL PUBLISHING COMPANY,
ST. PAUL, MINNESOTA
TEXT AND DISPLAY LINES ARE SET IN CALEDONIA

Library of Congress Cataloging in Publication Data
Main entry under title:
Wisconsin medicine.
Bibliography: pp. 185–200
Includes index.
Contents: Frontier medicine in the Territory of
Wisconsin / Peter T. Harstad — From horse and buggy
to automobile and telephone: medical practice in
Wisconsin, 1848–1930 / Guenter B. Risse — Sectarians
and scientists: alternatives to orthodox medicine / Eliz-
abeth Barnaby Keeney, Susan Eyrich Lederer, and Edmond
P. Minihan — [etc.]
1. Medicine — Wisconsin — History — Addresses, essays,
lectures. I. Numbers, Ronald L. II. Leavitt, Judith Walzer.
[DNLM: 1. History of medicine–Wisconsin. WZ 70 AW6 W8]
R357.W57   362.1'09775   80-52297
ISBN 0-299-08430-2   AACR2

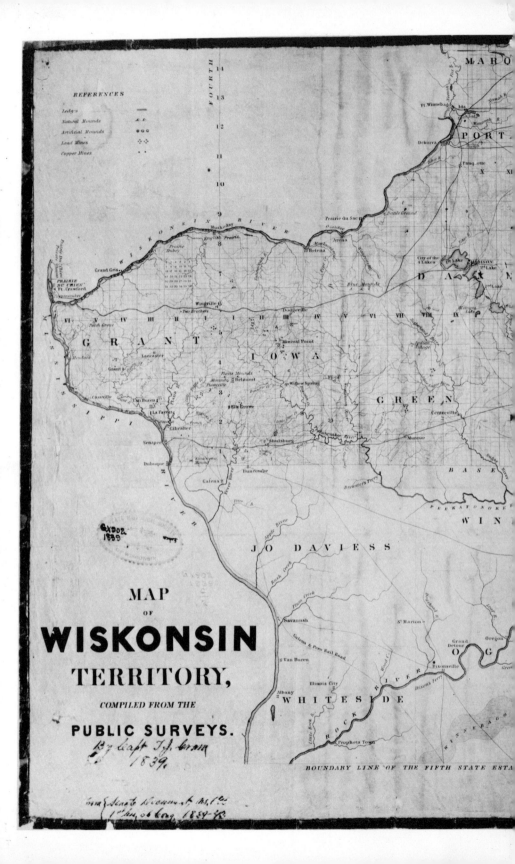

MAP

OF

WISKONSIN

TERRITORY,

COMPILED FROM THE

PUBLIC SURVEYS.

By Capt. T.J. Cram

1839.